Welcome to the ***"Greek Cookbook For Diabetics: 110+ Recipes and Meal Planning Resources for Diabetic-Friendly Greek Cooking."*** This cookbook is designed to bring the vibrant flavors of Greek cuisine to individuals managing diabetes, offering a collection of delicious recipes tailored to support blood sugar control and overall health.

In this book, you will discover a variety of traditional Greek dishes reimagined with a diabetic-friendly twist, allowing you to enjoy the rich flavors and wholesome ingredients of Mediterranean cooking while prioritizing your well-being. From hearty soups and salads to satisfying main courses and indulgent desserts, each recipe is carefully crafted to help you maintain stable blood sugar levels without compromising on taste.

In addition to the diverse range of recipes, this cookbook also provides valuable meal planning resources to assist you in creating balanced and nutritious meals that align with your dietary needs. Whether you are looking for quick and easy breakfast ideas, flavorful lunch and dinner options, or guilt-free snacks and beverages, this book has you covered.

Embrace the essence of Greek cuisine while taking charge of your health with the ***"Greek Cookbook For Diabetics."*** Explore the culinary delights of the Mediterranean and embark on a delicious journey towards better diabetes management and overall well-being.

1. Greek Salad (Horiatiki)

Ingredient:

- 1 cucumber, diced
- 2 tomatoes, diced
- 1 red onion, thinly sliced
- 1 green bell pepper, diced
- 1/2 cup pitted kalamata olives
- 1/2 cup crumbled feta cheese
- 2 tbsp olive oil
- 1 tbsp red wine vinegar
- 1 tsp dried oregano
- Salt and pepper to taste

Instructions:

1. In a large bowl, combine the diced cucumber, tomatoes, sliced onion, and diced bell pepper.

2. Add the pitted kalamata olives and crumbled feta cheese.

3. In a small bowl, whisk together the olive oil, red wine vinegar, and dried oregano. Season with salt and pepper to taste.

4. Pour the dressing over the salad and toss gently to coat.

5. Serve immediately or refrigerate until ready to serve.

This Greek salad is a great option for people with diabetes as it is low in carbs and high in healthy fats, fiber, and nutrients. The vegetables provide antioxidants, and the feta cheese adds a good source of protein. Enjoy this refreshing and flavorful salad as a main dish or a side.

2. Grilled Octopus

Ingredient:

• 1 lb octopus, cleaned and tentacles separated
• 2 tbsp olive oil
• 2 tbsp lemon juice
• 1 tsp dried oregano
• 1 tsp paprika
• Salt and pepper to taste

Instructions:

1. In a large pot, bring salted water to a boil. Add the octopus tentacles and cook for 30•40 minutes, until tender. Drain and let cool.

2. In a small bowl, whisk together the olive oil, lemon juice, oregano, and paprika. Season with salt and pepper.

3. Preheat grill or grill pan to medium•high heat.

4. Brush the octopus tentacles with the olive oil and lemon juice mixture.

5. Grill the octopus for 2•3 minutes per side, until charred and heated through.

6. Serve the grilled octopus warm, drizzled with any remaining olive oil and lemon juice mixture.

This grilled octopus dish is a great option for people with diabetes as it is low in carbs and high in protein. Octopus is also a good source of omega•3 fatty acids, which can help improve heart health. The lemon juice and oregano add flavor without adding extra calories or carbs.

Enjoy this delicious and healthy grilled octopus as a main dish or appetizer.

3. Grilled Fish (e.g., Sea Bass, Red Snapper)

Ingredient:

• 4 (6 oz) fillets of sea bass or red snapper
• 2 tbsp olive oil
• 1 tbsp lemon juice
• 1 tsp dried oregano
• 1 tsp garlic powder
• Salt and pepper to taste

Instructions:

1. Preheat grill or grill pan to medium•high heat.

2. In a small bowl, whisk together the olive oil, lemon juice, oregano, and garlic powder. Season with salt and pepper.

3. Pat the fish fillets dry with paper towels and brush both sides with the olive oil and lemon juice mixture.

4. Grill the fish for 3•4 minutes per side, or until it flakes easily with a fork and is cooked through.

5. Serve the grilled fish immediately, garnished with lemon wedges if desired.

This grilled fish recipe is a great option for people with diabetes as it is low in carbs and high in protein and healthy fats. Fish like sea bass and red snapper are also good sources of omega•3 fatty acids, which can help improve heart health.

The simple seasoning of lemon, oregano, and garlic adds flavor without adding extra calories or carbs. Serve this grilled fish with a side of roasted vegetables or a fresh salad for a complete and diabetes•friendly meal.

4. Lamb Kebabs (Souvlaki)

Ingredient:

- 1 lb lamb, cut into 1•inch cubes
- 1 red onion, cut into 1•inch pieces
- 1 red bell pepper, cut into 1•inch pieces
- 1 zucchini, cut into 1•inch pieces
- 2 tbsp olive oil
- 2 tbsp lemon juice
- 1 tsp dried oregano
- 1 tsp garlic powder
- Salt and pepper to taste

Instructions:

1. In a large bowl, combine the cubed lamb, onion, bell pepper, and zucchini.

2. In a small bowl, whisk together the olive oil, lemon juice, oregano, and garlic powder. Season with salt and pepper.

3. Pour the marinade over the lamb and vegetable mixture and toss to coat evenly.

4. Thread the marinated lamb and vegetables onto skewers, alternating the ingredients.

5. Preheat grill or grill pan to medium•high heat.

6. Grill the lamb kebabs for 8•10 minutes, turning occasionally, until the lamb is cooked through and the vegetables are tender.

7. Serve the grilled lamb kebabs immediately, garnished with additional lemon wedges if desired.

This lamb kebab recipe is a great option for people with diabetes as it is high in protein and low in carbs. The combination of lean lamb, fresh vegetables, and a simple lemon•oregano marinade provides a flavorful and healthy meal.

Serve the grilled lamb kebabs with a side of roasted vegetables or a fresh salad for a complete and diabetes•friendly meal.

5. Chicken Souvlaki

Ingredient:

• 1 lb boneless, skinless chicken breasts, cut into 1•inch cubes
• 2 tbsp olive oil
• 2 tbsp lemon juice
• 1 tsp dried oregano
• 1 tsp garlic powder
• Salt and pepper to taste
• 1 red onion, cut into 1•inch pieces
• 1 red bell pepper, cut into 1•inch pieces
• 1 zucchini, cut into 1•inch pieces

Instructions:

1. In a large bowl, combine the cubed chicken, olive oil, lemon juice, oregano, garlic powder, salt, and pepper. Toss to coat the chicken evenly.

2. Thread the marinated chicken, red onion, bell pepper, and zucchini onto skewers, alternating the ingredients.

3. Preheat grill or grill pan to medium•high heat.

4. Grill the chicken souvlaki skewers for 8•10 minutes, turning occasionally, until the chicken is cooked through and the vegetables are tender.

5. Serve the grilled chicken souvlaki immediately, garnished with additional lemon wedges if desired.

This chicken souvlaki recipe is a great option for people with diabetes as it is high in protein and low in carbs. The combination of lean chicken, fresh vegetables, and a simple lemon•oregano marinade provides a flavorful and healthy meal.

Serve the grilled chicken souvlaki with a side of roasted vegetables or a fresh salad for a complete and diabetes•friendly meal.

6. Shrimp Saganaki

Ingredient:

• 1 lb large shrimp, peeled and deveined
• 2 tbsp olive oil
• 1 onion, diced
• 3 cloves garlic, minced
• 1 (14 oz) can diced tomatoes
• 1/2 cup dry white wine
• 1 tsp dried oregano
• 1/4 tsp crushed red pepper flakes (optional)
• 1/2 cup crumbled feta cheese
• Salt and pepper to taste
• Chopped parsley for garnish

Instructions:

1. In a large skillet, heat the olive oil over medium heat. Add the diced onion and sauté for 3•4 minutes until translucent.

2. Add the minced garlic and sauté for an additional minute until fragrant.

3. Pour in the can of diced tomatoes and the white wine. Stir in the dried oregano and crushed red pepper flakes (if using).

4. Bring the mixture to a simmer and let it cook for 5•7 minutes, stirring occasionally, until the sauce has thickened slightly.

5. Add the peeled and deveined shrimp to the skillet and cook for 3•4 minutes, or until the shrimp are opaque and cooked through.

6. Remove the skillet from heat and sprinkle the crumbled feta cheese over the top.

7. Garnish with chopped parsley and serve immediately.

This Shrimp Saganaki dish is a great option for people with diabetes as it is low in carbs and high in protein and healthy fats. The tomato•based sauce and feta cheese provide a flavorful and satisfying meal.

Serve this dish with a side of roasted vegetables or a fresh salad for a complete and diabetes•friendly meal.

7. Stuffed Grape Leaves (Dolmades)

Ingredient:

• 1 jar (16 oz) grape leaves, drained and rinsed
• 1 lb ground lamb or ground turkey
• 1 cup cooked long•grain white rice
• 1 onion, finely chopped
• 2 cloves garlic, minced
• 1 tbsp fresh parsley, chopped
• 1 tsp dried mint
• 1 tsp lemon zest
• 1/4 cup lemon juice
• Salt and pepper to taste
• 2 cups low•sodium chicken or vegetable broth

Instructions:

1. In a large bowl, combine the ground lamb or turkey, cooked rice, chopped onion, minced garlic, parsley, dried mint, lemon zest, lemon juice, salt, and pepper. Mix well.

2. Lay a grape leaf shiny•side down on a flat surface. Place about 1•2 tablespoons of the filling near the stem end of the leaf. Fold the stem end over the filling, then fold the sides over and roll up tightly into a small bundle.

3. Arrange the stuffed grape leaves seam•side down in a large pot or baking dish. Pour the broth over the top.

4. Cover the pot or dish and simmer on the stove over low heat for 45•60 minutes, or until the grape leaves are tender and the filling is cooked through.

5. Serve the stuffed grape leaves warm, garnished with additional lemon wedges if desired.

This stuffed grape leaves recipe is a great option for people with diabetes as it is low in carbs and high in protein and healthy fats. The combination of ground meat, rice, and fresh herbs provides a flavorful and satisfying meal.

Enjoy these dolmades as a main dish or appetizer, paired with a fresh salad or roasted vegetables for a complete and diabetes•friendly meal.

8. Moussaka (can be made with lower·carb substitutions)

Ingredient:

- 1 lb ground lamb or ground beef
- 1 large eggplant, sliced into 1/2·inch rounds
- 1 onion, diced
- 3 cloves garlic, minced
- 1 (14 oz) can diced tomatoes
- 1 tsp dried oregano
- 1/2 tsp cinnamon

- Salt and pepper to taste
- Béchamel Sauce:
- 2 tbsp butter
- 2 tbsp almond flour or coconut flour
- 1 cup unsweetened almond milk
- 1/2 cup grated Parmesan cheese
- 2 eggs, lightly beaten
- 1/4 tsp nutmeg

Instructions:

1. Preheat oven to 375°F.

2. In a large skillet, cook the ground lamb or beef over medium heat until browned and crumbled. Drain any excess fat.

3. Add the diced onion and minced garlic to the skillet and sauté for 2·3 minutes until fragrant.

4. Stir in the diced tomatoes, oregano, cinnamon, salt, and pepper. Simmer for 10 minutes.

5. In a separate skillet, lightly sauté the eggplant slices until just tender, about 2·3 minutes per side. Set aside.

6. To make the béchamel sauce, melt the butter in a saucepan over medium heat. Whisk in the almond or coconut flour and cook for 1 minute. Gradually whisk in the almond milk and cook until thickened, about 5 minutes.

7. Remove the béchamel sauce from heat and stir in the Parmesan cheese, beaten eggs, and nutmeg. In a 9x13 inch baking dish, layer half of the eggplant slices, followed by the ground meat mixture, and then the remaining eggplant slices.

8. Pour the béchamel sauce over the top, spreading it evenly. Bake for 45·50 minutes, or until the top is golden brown and bubbly. Let the moussaka cool for 10·15 minutes before serving.

This moussaka recipe uses almond or coconut flour in the béchamel sauce to reduce the carb content, while still providing a creamy and flavorful topping. The eggplant and ground meat filling is a great source of protein and healthy fats.

9. Spanakopita (spinach pie with phyllo)

Ingredient:

• 1 lb fresh spinach, washed and chopped
• 1 onion, finely chopped
• 3 cloves garlic, minced
• 1 cup crumbled feta cheese
• 2 eggs, lightly beaten
• 1/4 cup grated Parmesan cheese
• 1 tsp dried dill
• 1/4 tsp nutmeg
• Salt and pepper to taste
• 8 sheets of low•carb or whole wheat phyllo dough, thawed if frozen

Filling:

1. In a large skillet, sauté the onion and garlic in a bit of olive oil until translucent.
2. Add the chopped spinach and cook until wilted, about 2•3 minutes. Drain any excess liquid.
3. In a bowl, mix the cooked spinach mixture with the feta, Parmesan, eggs, dill, nutmeg, salt, and pepper.

Assembly:

1. Preheat oven to 375°F.
2. Lay one sheet of phyllo dough in a 9x13 inch baking dish, brushing with a small amount of olive oil. Repeat with 3 more sheets, brushing each with oil.
3. Spread the spinach filling evenly over the phyllo.
4. Top with the remaining 4 sheets of phyllo, brushing each with oil.
5. Bake for 30•35 minutes, or until the phyllo is golden brown and crispy.
6. Let cool for 10 minutes before slicing and serving.

This spanakopita recipe uses low•carb or whole wheat phyllo dough to reduce the overall carb content, while still providing the flaky, crispy texture. The filling is high in protein and nutrients from the spinach, feta, and eggs, making it a great option for people with diabetes.

Serve this spanakopita as a main dish or appetizer, accompanied by a fresh salad or roasted vegetables for a complete and diabetes•friendly meal.

10. Tzatziki (cucumber yogurt dip)

Ingredient:

- 1 cup plain Greek yogurt (full•fat or low•fat)
- 1 cucumber, peeled, seeded, and grated
- 2 cloves garlic, minced
- 1 tbsp fresh lemon juice
- 1 tbsp chopped fresh dill
- 1/4 tsp salt
- 1/4 tsp black pepper

Instructions:

1. Place the grated cucumber in a clean kitchen towel or cheesecloth and squeeze out as much liquid as possible.

2. In a medium bowl, combine the strained cucumber, Greek yogurt, minced garlic, lemon juice, chopped dill, salt, and black pepper. Stir until well mixed.

3. Cover the tzatziki and refrigerate for at least 30 minutes to allow the flavors to meld.

4. Serve the tzatziki chilled, with pita bread, cucumber slices, or other low•carb dippers.

This tzatziki recipe is a great option for people with diabetes as it is low in carbs and high in protein and healthy fats from the Greek yogurt. The cucumber provides fiber and hydration, while the garlic, lemon, and dill add flavor without adding extra calories or carbs.

Tzatziki is a versatile dip that can be served as an appetizer or alongside grilled meats, roasted vegetables, or as a topping for dishes like grilled chicken or lamb.

Enjoy this refreshing and flavorful tzatziki as part of a diabetes•friendly Mediterranean•inspired meal.

11. Grilled Halloumi Cheese

Ingredient:

- 8 oz block of halloumi cheese, cut into 1/2•inch thick slices
- 1 tbsp olive oil
- 1 tbsp lemon juice
- 1 tsp dried oregano
- Salt and pepper to taste

Instructions:

1. Preheat grill or grill pan to medium•high heat.

2. In a shallow dish, whisk together the olive oil, lemon juice, and dried oregano. Season with salt and pepper.

3. Add the halloumi cheese slices to the dish and gently toss to coat both sides with the oil and lemon mixture.

4. Grill the halloumi slices for 2•3 minutes per side, or until grill marks appear and the cheese is slightly softened.

5. Carefully transfer the grilled halloumi slices to a serving plate.

6. Serve the grilled halloumi cheese warm, garnished with additional lemon wedges if desired.

This grilled halloumi cheese recipe is a great option for people with diabetes as it is low in carbs and high in protein and healthy fats. Halloumi is a semi•hard, brined cheese that has a high melting point, making it perfect for grilling.

The simple lemon and oregano marinade adds flavor without adding extra calories or carbs. Serve the grilled halloumi cheese as an appetizer or alongside a fresh salad or roasted vegetables for a complete and diabetes•friendly meal.

12. Roasted Eggplant Dip (Melitzanosalata)

Ingredient:

- 2 medium eggplants
- 2 cloves garlic, minced
- 2 tbsp olive oil
- 2 tbsp lemon juice
- 2 tbsp chopped fresh parsley
- 1 tbsp red wine vinegar
- 1/2 tsp salt
- 1/4 tsp black pepper

Instructions:

1. Preheat your oven to 400°F (200°C).

2. Prick the eggplants several times with a fork. Place them directly on the oven rack and roast for 30•40 minutes, until very soft. Allow to cool completely.

3. Once cooled, cut the eggplants in half lengthwise and scoop out the flesh into a food processor or blender. Discard the skins.

4. Add the minced garlic, olive oil, lemon juice, parsley, red wine vinegar, salt, and pepper to the food processor. Blend until smooth and creamy.

5. Transfer the dip to a serving bowl. Refrigerate for at least 30 minutes to allow the flavors to meld.

6. Serve the roasted eggplant dip with pita bread, crackers, or fresh vegetables.

This dip is a classic Greek appetizer that showcases the smoky, rich flavor of roasted eggplant. The lemon juice, garlic, and herbs provide a bright, refreshing contrast. Enjoy this healthy and flavorful dip!

13. Feta Cheese (in moderation)

Ingredient:

- 2 cups plain Greek yogurt
- 1 cup fresh berries (such as strawberries, blueberries, raspberries)
- 1/4 cup crumbled feta cheese
- 1/4 cup granola
- 1•2 tbsp honey (optional)

Instructions:

1. In a parfait glass or small bowl, layer the ingredients in the following order:
   - 1/4 cup Greek yogurt
   - 2•3 tbsp fresh berries
   - 1 tbsp crumbled feta cheese
   - 1 tbsp granola
   - Repeat the layers until you reach the top of the glass.

2. If desired, drizzle 1•2 teaspoons of honey over the top of the parfait.

3. Refrigerate the parfaits until ready to serve, at least 30 minutes.

4. Enjoy the parfaits chilled.

The feta cheese adds a savory, tangy element to balance the sweetness of the yogurt and fruit. The portion size of 1•2 tablespoons of feta keeps it in moderation, making this a suitable option for people with diabetes.

14. Greek Yogurt (unsweetened)

Ingredient:

• 2 cups plain Greek yogurt
• 1 cup fresh berries (such as strawberries, blueberries, raspberries)
• 1/2 cup granola
• 2 tbsp honey (optional)

Instructions:

1. In a parfait glass or small bowl, layer the ingredients in the following order:
   • 1/4 cup Greek yogurt
   • 1/4 cup fresh berries
   • 1•2 tbsp granola
   • Repeat the layers until you reach the top of the glass.

2. If desired, drizzle 1•2 teaspoons of honey over the top of the parfait.

3. Refrigerate the parfaits until ready to serve, at least 30 minutes.

4. Enjoy the parfaits chilled. The Greek yogurt provides protein, the berries add antioxidants and fiber, and the granola gives a nice crunch.

You can easily customize the parfaits by using different types of fruit, nuts, seeds, or even a sprinkle of cinnamon or cocoa powder on top. The key is to create layers of creamy yogurt, sweet fruit, and crunchy granola. This makes for a healthy, satisfying breakfast or snack.

15. Lentil Soup (Fakes Soupa)

Ingredient:

- 1 cup dried brown or green lentils, rinsed
- 6 cups low•sodium vegetable or chicken broth
- 1 onion, diced
- 2 carrots, peeled and diced
- 2 celery stalks, diced
- 3 cloves garlic, minced
- 2 tbsp tomato paste
- 1 tsp dried oregano
- 1 bay leaf
- 1/4 tsp ground black pepper
- 2 tbsp lemon juice
- 2 tbsp chopped fresh parsley

Instructions:

1. In a large pot, combine the lentils and broth. Bring to a boil over high heat.

2. Reduce heat to medium•low, cover and simmer for 20•25 minutes, until the lentils are tender.

3. Add the onion, carrots, celery, and garlic. Simmer for an additional 10•15 minutes, until the vegetables are soft.

4. Stir in the tomato paste, oregano, bay leaf, and black pepper. Simmer for 5 more minutes.

5. Remove the bay leaf. Stir in the lemon juice and parsley.

6. Serve the lentil soup hot. Garnish with additional parsley if desired.

This lentil soup is high in fiber, protein, and complex carbohydrates, making it a great option for people with diabetes. The vegetables and herbs add flavor without adding too many carbs. Enjoy this hearty, nutritious soup!

16. Baked Chicken with Herbs

Ingredient:

• 4 boneless, skinless chicken breasts
• 2 tbsp olive oil
• 1 tsp dried oregano
• 1 tsp dried thyme
• 1 tsp garlic powder
• 1/2 tsp salt
• 1/4 tsp black pepper

Instructions:

1. Preheat your oven to 400°F (200°C).

2. In a small bowl, combine the olive oil, oregano, thyme, garlic powder, salt, and black pepper. Mix well.

3. Place the chicken breasts in a baking dish or on a rimmed baking sheet. Brush or rub the herb mixture evenly over the top and sides of the chicken.

4. Bake the chicken for 25•30 minutes, or until it reaches an internal temperature of 165°F (75°C) when measured with a meat thermometer.

5. Remove the baked chicken from the oven and let it rest for 5 minutes before serving.

This baked chicken recipe is a great option for people with diabetes as it is low in carbs and high in protein. The combination of herbs and spices adds flavor without adding extra calories or carbs.

Serve the baked chicken with a side of roasted vegetables or a fresh salad for a complete and diabetes•friendly meal. You can also use the leftover chicken in other dishes, such as salads or wraps, throughout the week.

17. Baked Fish with Lemon and Herbs

Ingredient:

- 1 lb white fish fillets (such as cod, tilapia, or halibut)
- 2 tbsp olive oil
- 2 tbsp freshly squeezed lemon juice
- 2 tsp dried oregano
- 1 tsp dried thyme
- 1 tsp garlic powder
- 1/2 tsp salt
- 1/4 tsp black pepper
- 1 lemon, sliced
- 2 tbsp chopped fresh parsley

Instructions:

1. Preheat your oven to 400°F (200°C). Lightly grease a baking dish or line it with parchment paper.

2. Pat the fish fillets dry with paper towels and place them in the prepared baking dish.

3. In a small bowl, whisk together the olive oil, lemon juice, oregano, thyme, garlic powder, salt, and pepper.

4. Drizzle the lemon•herb mixture over the fish fillets, making sure to coat them evenly.

5. Arrange the lemon slices on top of the fish.

6. Bake for 15•20 minutes, or until the fish is cooked through and flakes easily with a fork.

7. Remove the baked fish from the oven and sprinkle with the chopped fresh parsley.

8. Serve the fish immediately, with the lemon slices and any pan juices spooned over the top.

This baked fish dish is simple, yet full of bright, Mediterranean flavors from the lemon, herbs, and garlic. It's a healthy, low•carb option that pairs well with roasted vegetables or a fresh salad. Enjoy!

18. Grilled Vegetables

Ingredient:

- 1 zucchini, sliced into 1/2·inch thick rounds
- 1 yellow squash, sliced into 1/2·inch thick rounds
- 1 red bell pepper, cut into 1·inch pieces
- 1 yellow onion, sliced into 1/2·inch thick rounds
- 8 oz mushrooms, halved or quartered
- 2 tbsp olive oil
- 1 tsp dried oregano
- 1 tsp dried basil
- 1/2 tsp salt
- 1/4 tsp black pepper

Instructions:

1. Preheat your grill or grill pan to medium·high heat.

2. In a large bowl, toss the sliced vegetables with the olive oil, oregano, basil, salt, and pepper until evenly coated.

3. Arrange the vegetables in a single layer on the hot grill or grill pan. Cook for 4·5 minutes per side, or until they are tender and have nice grill marks.

4. Use tongs to transfer the grilled vegetables to a serving platter.

5. Serve the grilled vegetables warm, as a side dish or as part of a larger meal.

Tips:
- You can use any combination of vegetables you like, such as eggplant, asparagus, or cherry tomatoes.
- Soak wooden skewers in water for 30 minutes before threading vegetables onto them for easy turning on the grill.
- Brush the vegetables with a bit of olive oil or balsamic vinegar after grilling for extra flavor.

This simple grilled vegetable recipe is a great way to enjoy the natural sweetness and texture of fresh produce. It's a healthy, low·carb side dish that pairs well with grilled meats, fish, or as part of a Mediterranean·inspired meal.

19. Greek Chicken Salad

Ingredient:

- 2 boneless, skinless chicken breasts, grilled and diced
- 1 cup cherry tomatoes, halved
- 1 cucumber, diced
- 1/2 red onion, thinly sliced
- 1/2 cup crumbled feta cheese
- 1/4 cup kalamata olives, pitted and halved
- 2 tbsp chopped fresh parsley
- 2 tbsp chopped fresh dill
- 2 tbsp olive oil
- 1 tbsp red wine vinegar
- 1 tbsp lemon juice
- 1 tsp dried oregano
- 1/4 tsp salt
- 1/4 tsp black pepper

Instructions:

1. In a large bowl, combine the diced grilled chicken, cherry tomatoes, cucumber, red onion, feta cheese, olives, parsley, and dill.

2. In a small bowl, whisk together the olive oil, red wine vinegar, lemon juice, oregano, salt, and pepper.

3. Pour the dressing over the salad and toss gently to coat.

4. Refrigerate the Greek chicken salad for at least 30 minutes to allow the flavors to meld.

5. Serve the salad chilled or at room temperature. It can be served on a bed of greens, stuffed into pita pockets, or enjoyed on its own.

This Greek chicken salad is packed with fresh vegetables, protein•rich chicken, and the bold flavors of feta, olives, and Mediterranean herbs. It's a light, refreshing, and healthy main dish or side salad. Adjust the amounts of ingredients to your taste preferences.

20. Lemon Garlic Shrimp

Ingredient:

- 1 lb large shrimp, peeled and deveined
- 3 tbsp olive oil
- 4 cloves garlic, minced
- 1 tbsp lemon zest
- 2 tbsp freshly squeezed lemon juice
- 1/4 tsp red pepper flakes (optional)
- 1/4 tsp salt
- 1/4 tsp black pepper
- 2 tbsp chopped fresh parsley

Instructions:

1. In a large skillet, heat the olive oil over medium•high heat.

2. Add the minced garlic and sauté for 1 minute, until fragrant.

3. Add the shrimp, lemon zest, lemon juice, red pepper flakes (if using), salt, and black pepper. Toss to coat the shrimp evenly.

4. Cook the shrimp for 2•3 minutes per side, or until they are opaque and cooked through.

5. Remove the skillet from the heat and stir in the chopped fresh parsley.

6. Serve the lemon garlic shrimp immediately, while hot. It pairs well with steamed vegetables, pasta, or crusty bread.

Tips:
- Use large, high•quality shrimp for the best texture and flavor.
- Adjust the amount of red pepper flakes to your desired level of spiciness.
- Garnish with additional lemon wedges, if desired.

This quick and easy lemon garlic shrimp dish is bursting with bright, zesty flavors. The shrimp cooks up quickly, making it a great option for a weeknight meal. Enjoy this healthy, low•carb seafood dish!

21. Greek Frittata

Ingredient:

• 8 eggs
• 1/4 cup milk
• 1/4 tsp salt
• 1/4 tsp black pepper
• 2 tbsp olive oil
• 1 onion, diced
• 2 cloves garlic, minced
• 1 cup cherry tomatoes, halved
• 1 cup baby spinach leaves
• 1/2 cup crumbled feta cheese
• 2 tbsp chopped fresh parsley

Instructions:

1. Preheat your oven to 375°F (190°C).

2. In a medium bowl, whisk together the eggs, milk, salt, and black pepper. Set aside.

3. In a 9•inch oven•safe skillet (such as cast iron), heat the olive oil over medium heat.

4. Add the diced onion and sauté for 3•4 minutes, until translucent.

5. Stir in the minced garlic and cook for 1 minute, until fragrant.

6. Add the halved cherry tomatoes and baby spinach leaves. Cook for 2•3 minutes, until the spinach is wilted.

7. Pour the egg mixture over the vegetables in the skillet. Sprinkle the crumbled feta cheese evenly over the top.

8. Transfer the skillet to the preheated oven and bake for 15•20 minutes, or until the frittata is set and the edges are lightly golden. Remove the Greek frittata from the oven and let it cool for a few minutes.

10. Sprinkle the chopped fresh parsley over the top before serving. Cut the frittata into wedges and serve warm or at room temperature.

This Greek•inspired frittata is a delicious and easy•to•make breakfast or brunch dish. The combination of eggs, feta, tomatoes, and spinach creates a flavorful and nutritious meal. Enjoy it on its own or with a side of pita bread or a fresh Greek salad

22. Baked Feta with Tomatoes and Olives

Ingredient:

• 8 oz block of feta cheese
• 1 cup cherry tomatoes, halved
• 1/2 cup pitted kalamata olives, halved
• 2 cloves garlic, minced
• 2 tbsp olive oil
• 1 tsp dried oregano
• 1/4 tsp red pepper flakes (optional)
• Salt and black pepper to taste
• Fresh basil leaves for garnish (optional)

Instructions:

1. Preheat your oven to 400°F (200°C). Lightly grease a small baking dish or oven•safe skillet.

2. Place the block of feta cheese in the center of the prepared baking dish.

3. In a bowl, combine the halved cherry tomatoes, halved kalamata olives, minced garlic, olive oil, dried oregano, and red pepper flakes (if using). Season with salt and black pepper to taste.

4. Spoon the tomato•olive mixture around the feta cheese, making sure to cover the top and sides of the cheese.

5. Bake for 15•20 minutes, or until the feta is softened and the tomatoes are slightly blistered.

6. Remove the baked feta from the oven and let it cool for a few minutes.

7. Garnish the baked feta with fresh basil leaves, if desired. Serve the warm baked feta immediately, with crusty bread or pita for dipping in the flavorful juices.

This simple, yet impressive baked feta dish is a classic Greek appetizer. The combination of creamy feta, juicy tomatoes, and briny olives creates a delicious and easy•to•prepare Mediterranean•inspired treat. Adjust the amount of red pepper flakes to your desired level of spiciness.

23. Greek·Style Meatballs (Keftedes)

Ingredient:

- 1 lb ground beef or lamb (or a combination)
- 1 onion, finely chopped
- 3 cloves garlic, minced
- 1/2 cup breadcrumbs
- 1 egg, lightly beaten
- 2 tbsp chopped fresh parsley
- 1 tsp dried oregano
- 1 tsp ground cinnamon
- 1/2 tsp ground allspice
- 1/2 tsp salt
- 1/4 tsp black pepper
- 2 tbsp olive oil for frying

Instructions:

1. In a large bowl, combine the ground meat, onion, garlic, breadcrumbs, egg, parsley, oregano, cinnamon, allspice, salt, and pepper. Mix well until all the ingredients are evenly distributed.

2. Using your hands, form the mixture into small, golf ball·sized meatballs.

3. In a large skillet, heat the olive oil over medium·high heat.

4. Working in batches, carefully add the meatballs to the hot oil and fry for 2·3 minutes per side, until they are golden brown on the outside and cooked through.

5. Transfer the cooked meatballs to a paper towel·lined plate to drain any excess oil.

6. Serve the Greek·style meatballs warm, either on their own or with tzatziki sauce, pita bread, and a Greek salad.

Tips:
- For a lighter version, you can bake the meatballs in the oven at 400°F (200°C) for 15·20 minutes instead of frying.
- Adjust the spices to your taste preferences, adding more or less cinnamon and allspice as desired.
- Make the meatballs ahead of time and reheat them before serving.

These flavorful Greek·style meatballs are a delicious and versatile dish that can be enjoyed as an appetizer or as part of a larger Greek·inspired meal

24. Greek•Style Baked Cod

Ingredient:

• 1 lb cod fillets, cut into 4 portions
• 2 tbsp olive oil
• 2 tbsp lemon juice
• 2 cloves garlic, minced
• 1 tsp dried oregano
• 1/2 tsp dried thyme
• 1/4 tsp salt
• 1/4 tsp black pepper
• 1 cup cherry tomatoes, halved
• 1/2 cup crumbled feta cheese
• 2 tbsp chopped fresh parsley

Instructions:

1. Preheat your oven to 400°F (200°C). Lightly grease a baking dish or line it with parchment paper.

2. Place the cod fillets in the prepared baking dish.

3. In a small bowl, whisk together the olive oil, lemon juice, garlic, oregano, thyme, salt, and pepper.

4. Drizzle the lemon•herb mixture over the cod fillets, making sure to coat them evenly.

5. Scatter the halved cherry tomatoes around the cod.

6. Sprinkle the crumbled feta cheese over the top.

7. Bake for 15•20 minutes, or until the cod is cooked through and flakes easily with a fork.

8. Remove the baked cod from the oven and sprinkle with the chopped fresh parsley.

9. Serve the Greek•style baked cod immediately, with the tomatoes and pan juices spooned over the top.

This baked cod dish is a healthy and flavorful way to enjoy seafood. The lemon, herbs, and feta cheese give it a distinctly Greek flavor profile. Serve it with roasted vegetables, a Greek salad, or lemon•garlic roasted potatoes for a complete Mediterranean•inspired meal

25. Stewed Green Beans (Fasolakia)

Ingredient:

- 1 lb green beans, trimmed and cut into 1•inch pieces
- 2 tbsp olive oil
- 1 onion, diced
- 3 cloves garlic, minced
- 1 cup diced tomatoes (canned or fresh)
- 1 cup low•sodium vegetable or chicken broth
- 1 tsp dried oregano
- 1/2 tsp salt
- 1/4 tsp black pepper
- 2 tbsp chopped fresh parsley

Instructions:

1. In a large skillet or Dutch oven, heat the olive oil over medium heat.

2. Add the diced onion and sauté for 3•4 minutes, until translucent.

3. Stir in the minced garlic and cook for 1 minute, until fragrant.

4. Add the cut green beans, diced tomatoes, vegetable broth, oregano, salt, and pepper. Stir to combine.

5. Bring the mixture to a boil, then reduce heat to low, cover, and simmer for 20•25 minutes, stirring occasionally, until the green beans are very tender.

6. Remove the lid and continue simmering for 5 more minutes to allow the sauce to thicken slightly.

7. Stir in the chopped fresh parsley just before serving.

8. Serve the stewed green beans warm, as a side dish. They pair well with grilled or roasted meats, fish, or as part of a Greek•inspired meal.

This classic Greek dish showcases the simple, comforting flavors of tender green beans simmered in a tomato•based sauce. The long cooking time allows the flavors to meld together beautifully. Adjust the seasoning to your taste preferences.

26. Lamb Chops

Ingredient:

• 8 lamb chops (about 1•inch thick)
• 2 tbsp olive oil
• 2 tsp dried oregano
• 1 tsp dried thyme
• 1 tsp garlic powder
• 1 tsp salt
• 1/2 tsp black pepper

Instructions:

1. Pat the lamb chops dry with paper towels and place them in a shallow baking dish or large resealable plastic bag.

2. In a small bowl, mix together the olive oil, oregano, thyme, garlic powder, salt, and black pepper.

3. Pour the marinade over the lamb chops and turn to coat them evenly. Cover and refrigerate for 30 minutes to 1 hour.

4. Preheat your grill or grill pan to medium•high heat.

5. Remove the lamb chops from the marinade and place them on the hot grill. Grill for 3•4 minutes per side, or until they reach your desired doneness.

6. Transfer the grilled lamb chops to a serving platter and let them rest for 5 minutes before serving.

Serving Suggestions:
• Serve the grilled lamb chops with roasted vegetables, a Greek salad, or lemon•garlic roasted potatoes.
• Garnish with fresh chopped parsley or mint.
• Squeeze a little fresh lemon juice over the top just before serving.

This simple grilled lamb chop recipe allows the natural flavors of the meat to shine, with a boost from the Mediterranean•inspired herbs and spices. Adjust the cooking time based on your preferred level of doneness. Enjoy this delicious and healthy lamb dish!

27. Greek•Style Roasted Chicken

Ingredient:

• 1 whole chicken (3•4 lbs), cut into 8 pieces (breasts, thighs, legs, wings)
• 2 tbsp olive oil
• 2 tbsp lemon juice
• 3 cloves garlic, minced
• 1 tsp dried oregano
• 1 tsp dried thyme
• 1/2 tsp salt
• 1/4 tsp black pepper
• 1 lemon, sliced
• 1 onion, sliced
• 2 sprigs fresh rosemary

Instructions:

1. Preheat your oven to 400°F (200°C). Lightly grease a large baking dish or rimmed baking sheet.

2. In a large bowl, combine the olive oil, lemon juice, minced garlic, oregano, thyme, salt, and black pepper. Add the chicken pieces and toss to coat them evenly with the marinade.

3. Arrange the marinated chicken pieces in the prepared baking dish or on the baking sheet. Scatter the lemon slices, onion slices, and rosemary sprigs around the chicken.

4. Roast the chicken in the preheated oven for 45•55 minutes, or until the chicken is cooked through and the juices run clear when pierced with a fork.

5. Baste the chicken with the pan juices halfway through the cooking time.

6. Remove the roasted chicken from the oven and let it rest for 5•10 minutes before serving.

7. Serve the Greek•style roasted chicken warm, with the roasted lemon and onion slices spooned over the top. Garnish with additional fresh rosemary, if desired.

This flavorful Greek•inspired roasted chicken dish is a simple and delicious main course. The lemon, garlic, and herbs create a bright, Mediterranean flavor profile that pairs well with roasted vegetables or a fresh Greek salad.

28. Greek Egg Drop Soup (Avgolemono)

Ingredient:

• 4 cups low•sodium chicken or vegetable broth
• 1/3 cup uncooked white rice
• 2 eggs
• 2 tbsp fresh lemon juice
• 1 tsp grated lemon zest
• 2 tbsp chopped fresh dill
• Salt and pepper to taste

Instructions:

1. In a medium saucepan, bring the broth to a boil over high heat. Add the uncooked rice, reduce heat to medium•low, and simmer for 15•20 minutes, until the rice is tender.

2. In a small bowl, whisk together the eggs and lemon juice until well combined.

3. Once the rice is cooked, reduce the heat to low. Slowly drizzle the egg•lemon mixture into the hot broth, whisking constantly, to create the "egg drop" effect.

4. Remove the saucepan from the heat and stir in the grated lemon zest and chopped fresh dill.

5. Season the avgolemono soup with salt and pepper to taste.

6. Serve the Greek egg drop soup warm, garnished with additional dill if desired.

Tips:
• For a thicker soup, use short•grain rice like arborio or sushi rice.
• Adjust the amount of lemon juice to your taste preference.
• You can also add shredded chicken or cooked orzo pasta to the soup for extra heartiness.

This traditional Greek soup, known as avgolemono, is a comforting and tangy dish that showcases the bright flavors of lemon and dill. The egg•lemon mixture creates a velvety texture that complements the rice and broth. Enjoy this simple, yet flavorful soup as a light meal or appetizer.

29. Greek Cauliflower Rice Pilaf

Ingredient:

• 1 head of cauliflower, cut into florets
• 2 tbsp olive oil
• 1 onion, diced
• 2 cloves garlic, minced
• 1 cup diced tomatoes (canned or fresh)
• 1/2 cup crumbled feta cheese
• 2 tbsp chopped fresh parsley
• 1 tsp dried oregano
• 1/4 tsp salt
• 1/4 tsp black pepper

Instructions:

1. In a food processor, pulse the cauliflower florets until they resemble the texture of rice. Set aside.

2. In a large skillet, heat the olive oil over medium heat. Add the diced onion and sauté for 3•4 minutes, until translucent.

3. Stir in the minced garlic and cook for 1 minute, until fragrant.

4. Add the riced cauliflower to the skillet and sauté for 5•7 minutes, stirring occasionally, until the cauliflower is tender.

5. Stir in the diced tomatoes, crumbled feta cheese, chopped parsley, dried oregano, salt, and black pepper. Cook for an additional 2•3 minutes, until the flavors are combined.

6. Remove the Greek cauliflower rice pilaf from the heat and serve warm.

Variations:
• For extra flavor, add a splash of lemon juice or a drizzle of balsamic glaze.
• Stir in some cooked chickpeas or diced grilled chicken for a more substantial meal.
• Top with toasted pine nuts or sliced olives for additional texture and flavor.

This Greek•inspired cauliflower rice pilaf is a healthy, low•carb alternative to traditional rice dishes. The combination of riced cauliflower, tomatoes, feta, and Mediterranean herbs creates a delicious and nutritious side dish or vegetarian main course.

30. Greek•Style Zucchini

Ingredient:

- 2 lbs zucchini, sliced into 1/2•inch thick rounds
- 2 tbsp olive oil
- 1 onion, diced
- 3 cloves garlic, minced
- 1 cup diced tomatoes (canned or fresh)
- 1/4 cup crumbled feta cheese
- 2 tbsp chopped fresh parsley
- 1 tsp dried oregano
- 1/4 tsp salt
- 1/4 tsp black pepper

Instructions:

1. Preheat your oven to 400°F (200°C). Lightly grease a large baking sheet or casserole dish.

2. Arrange the sliced zucchini rounds in a single layer on the prepared baking sheet or dish.

3. In a skillet, heat the olive oil over medium heat. Add the diced onion and sauté for 3•4 minutes, until translucent.

4. Stir in the minced garlic and cook for 1 minute, until fragrant.

5. Add the diced tomatoes to the skillet and cook for 2•3 minutes, until slightly thickened.

6. Remove the skillet from the heat and stir in the crumbled feta cheese, chopped parsley, dried oregano, salt, and black pepper.

7. Spoon the tomato•feta mixture evenly over the sliced zucchini.

8. Bake the Greek•style zucchini in the preheated oven for 20•25 minutes, until the zucchini is tender and the topping is lightly browned. Serve the baked zucchini warm, garnished with additional parsley if desired.

This simple, yet flavorful Greek•inspired zucchini dish is a great way to enjoy summer produce. The combination of zucchini, tomatoes, feta, and herbs creates a delicious and healthy side dish. Adjust the seasoning to your taste preferences

31. Greek•Style Spinach and Cheese Pie

Ingredient:

• 1 lb fresh spinach, washed and chopped
• 1 onion, finely chopped
• 3 cloves garlic, minced
• 1 cup crumbled feta cheese
• 1/2 cup ricotta cheese
• 2 eggs, lightly beaten
• 1/4 cup chopped fresh dill
• 1/4 cup chopped fresh parsley
• 1 tsp dried oregano
• 1/4 tsp nutmeg
• 1/4 tsp salt
• 1/8 tsp black pepper
• 8 sheets phyllo dough, thawed if frozen
• 4 tbsp melted butter or olive oil

Instructions:

1. Preheat your oven to 375°F (190°C). Grease a 9•inch pie dish or baking pan.

2. In a large skillet, sauté the chopped onion in a bit of olive oil over medium heat until translucent, about 5 minutes. Add the minced garlic and cook for 1 minute more.

3. Add the chopped spinach to the skillet and cook, stirring frequently, until the spinach is wilted and any excess moisture has evaporated, about 5•7 minutes. Remove from heat and let cool slightly.

4. In a large bowl, combine the sautéed spinach mixture, feta cheese, ricotta cheese, beaten eggs, dill, parsley, oregano, nutmeg, salt, and pepper. Mix well.

5. Lay one sheet of phyllo dough in the prepared baking dish, allowing the edges to hang over the sides. Brush the phyllo with melted butter or olive oil. Repeat with 3 more sheets of phyllo, brushing each layer with butter/oil.

6. Spread the spinach and cheese filling evenly over the phyllo base. Top the filling with the remaining 4 sheets of phyllo, brushing each layer with butter/oil.

8. Fold the overhanging phyllo dough over the top of the pie to create a rustic, layered effect.Bake the spanakopita for 35•40 minutes, until the phyllo is golden brown and crispy. Let the pie cool for 10•15 minutes before slicing and serving.

32. Grilled Greek Chicken Wings

Ingredient:

- 2 lbs chicken wings, drumettes and flats separated
- 2 tbsp olive oil
- 2 tbsp lemon juice
- 2 tsp dried oregano
- 1 tsp garlic powder
- 1/2 tsp salt
- 1/4 tsp black pepper
- 2 tbsp chopped fresh parsley (for garnish)

Instructions:

1. In a large resealable bag or bowl, combine the chicken wings, olive oil, lemon juice, oregano, garlic powder, salt, and black pepper. Toss to coat the wings evenly.

2. Cover and marinate the chicken wings in the refrigerator for 30 minutes to 1 hour.

3. Preheat your grill or grill pan to medium•high heat.

4. Remove the chicken wings from the marinade and discard any remaining marinade.

5. Grill the chicken wings for 15•20 minutes, turning occasionally, until they are cooked through and the skin is crispy.

6. Transfer the grilled Greek chicken wings to a serving platter and garnish with the chopped fresh parsley.

7. Serve the wings warm.

This grilled Greek chicken wing recipe is a great option for people with diabetes as it is low in carbs and high in protein. The lemon, oregano, and garlic provide a flavorful Mediterranean twist without adding any sugars.

You can serve these wings as an appetizer or a main dish, accompanied by a fresh Greek salad or roasted vegetables for a complete and healthy meal.

33. Greek Cabbage Rolls

Ingredient:

- 1 medium head green cabbage
- 1 lb ground beef or lamb
- 1 onion, finely chopped
- 2 cloves garlic, minced
- 1/2 cup uncooked long•grain rice
- 2 tbsp chopped fresh parsley
- 1 tsp dried oregano

- 1/2 tsp ground cinnamon
- 1/4 tsp ground allspice
- 1/4 tsp salt
- 1/4 tsp black pepper
- 1 (14 oz) can diced tomatoes
- 1 cup vegetable or chicken broth
- 2 tbsp lemon juice
- Olive oil for drizzling

Instructions:

1. Bring a large pot of water to a boil. Carefully add the whole head of cabbage and cook for 2•3 minutes, until the outer leaves are softened. Remove the cabbage and let it cool slightly.

2. Carefully peel off the softened cabbage leaves, keeping them intact. You should have about 12•14 leaves.

3. In a large bowl, combine the ground meat, onion, garlic, uncooked rice, parsley, oregano, cinnamon, allspice, salt, and pepper. Mix well.

4. Place about 2•3 tablespoons of the meat mixture onto the center of each cabbage leaf. Fold the sides of the leaf over the filling, then roll up tightly to enclose the filling.

5. Arrange the stuffed cabbage rolls seam•side down in a large baking dish or Dutch oven. Pour the diced tomatoes and broth over the rolls.

6. Drizzle the tops of the rolls with a little olive oil and sprinkle with the lemon juice.

7. Cover the dish and bake at 350°F (175°C) for 1 to 1 1/2 hours, until the cabbage is tender and the filling is cooked through. Serve the Greek cabbage rolls warm, with the tomato•based sauce spooned over the top.

These traditional Greek cabbage rolls are a hearty and flavorful dish. The combination of ground meat, rice, and Mediterranean spices makes for a delicious and satisfying meal.

34. Greek•Style Grilled Pork

Ingredient:

• 1 lb pork tenderloin, trimmed of any visible fat
• 2 tbsp olive oil
• 2 tbsp lemon juice
• 1 tsp dried oregano
• 1 tsp garlic powder
• 1/2 tsp salt
• 1/4 tsp black pepper

Instructions:

1. In a shallow dish, combine the olive oil, lemon juice, oregano, garlic powder, salt, and pepper. Add the pork tenderloin and turn to coat both sides with the marinade. Cover and refrigerate for 30 minutes to 1 hour.

2. Preheat grill or grill pan to medium•high heat.

3. Grill the pork for 12•15 minutes, turning occasionally, until the internal temperature reaches 145°F.

4. Transfer the pork to a cutting board and let rest for 5 minutes before slicing.

5. Slice the pork into 1/2•inch thick slices and serve.

Nutritional Information (per serving):
Calories: 180
Total Fat: 7g
Saturated Fat: 2g
Carbohydrates: 1g
Fiber: 0g
Protein: 26g

This Greek•style grilled pork is a lean, flavorful option that is suitable for people with diabetes. The marinade adds lots of flavor without adding a lot of extra calories or carbs. Pair it with a side salad or roasted vegetables for a complete, diabetes•friendly meal.

35. Greek Green Salad with Lemon Dressing

Ingredient:

- 6 cups mixed greens (such as romaine, spinach, and arugula)
- 1 cucumber, sliced
- 1 cup cherry tomatoes, halved
- 1/2 red onion, thinly sliced
- 1/2 cup crumbled feta cheese
- 1/4 cup kalamata olives, pitted and halved
- 2 tbsp chopped fresh parsley
- 2 tbsp fresh lemon juice
- 1 tbsp olive oil
- 1 tsp Dijon mustard
- 1 tsp dried oregano
- 1/4 tsp salt
- 1/4 tsp black pepper

Instructions:

1. In a large salad bowl, combine the mixed greens, sliced cucumber, cherry tomatoes, red onion, crumbled feta cheese, and kalamata olives.

2. In a small bowl, whisk together the lemon juice, olive oil, Dijon mustard, dried oregano, salt, and black pepper to make the dressing.

3. Drizzle the lemon dressing over the salad and toss gently to coat.

4. Sprinkle the chopped fresh parsley over the top of the salad.

5. Serve the Greek green salad immediately.

This salad is a great option for people with diabetes as it is low in carbs and high in fiber, vitamins, and healthy fats from the olive oil and feta cheese. The lemon dressing provides a bright, tangy flavor without adding any additional sugars.

You can adjust the amounts of the ingredients to your taste preferences. This salad pairs well with grilled chicken, fish, or as a side dish to a Mediterranean•inspired meal.

36. Greek•Style Beef Stew

Ingredient:

- 1 lb lean beef stew meat, cut into 1•inch cubes
- 2 tbsp olive oil
- 1 onion, diced
- 3 cloves garlic, minced
- 1 tsp dried oregano
- 1 tsp dried thyme
- 1/2 tsp cinnamon
- 1/4 tsp ground cloves
- 1 (14.5 oz) can diced tomatoes
- 2 cups low•sodium beef broth
- 2 medium potatoes, peeled and cubed
- 2 carrots, peeled and sliced
- 1 cup frozen green beans
- 2 tbsp lemon juice
- 2 tbsp chopped fresh parsley
- 1/4 cup crumbled feta cheese

Instructions:

1. In a large pot or Dutch oven, heat the olive oil over medium•high heat. Add the beef cubes and brown on all sides, about 5 minutes total. Remove beef and set aside.

2. Add the onion to the pot and cook for 3•4 minutes until softened. Add the garlic and cook for 1 minute more.

3. Stir in the oregano, thyme, cinnamon, and cloves. Cook for 1 minute to toast the spices.

4. Pour in the diced tomatoes and beef broth. Add the browned beef back to the pot along with the potatoes and carrots.

5. Bring the stew to a boil, then reduce heat and simmer for 45•60 minutes, until the beef and vegetables are tender. Stir in the frozen green beans and lemon juice. Cook for 5 more minutes.

7. Remove from heat and stir in the chopped parsley. Serve the Greek•style beef stew warm, topped with crumbled feta cheese.

This hearty Greek•style beef stew is a diabetes•friendly meal. The lean beef, vegetables, and spices provide fiber, protein, and nutrients without a lot of extra carbs or calories. Adjust the amount of feta cheese to control the sodium content if needed.

37. Greek•Style Roasted Vegetables

Ingredient:

- 1 lb zucchini, cut into 1•inch pieces
- 1 lb eggplant, cut into 1•inch pieces
- 1 lb bell peppers, cut into 1•inch pieces
- 1 red onion, cut into 1•inch wedges
- 3 tbsp olive oil
- 2 tsp dried oregano
- 1 tsp garlic powder
- 1/2 tsp salt
- 1/4 tsp black pepper
- 2 tbsp crumbled feta cheese
- 2 tbsp chopped fresh parsley

Instructions:

1. Preheat oven to 400°F. Line a large baking sheet with parchment paper.

2. In a large bowl, toss the zucchini, eggplant, bell peppers, and onion with the olive oil, oregano, garlic powder, salt, and pepper until evenly coated.

3. Spread the vegetables in a single layer on the prepared baking sheet.

4. Roast for 25•30 minutes, stirring halfway, until the vegetables are tender and lightly browned.

5. Transfer the roasted vegetables to a serving dish. Sprinkle the crumbled feta cheese and chopped parsley over the top.

6. Serve the Greek•style roasted vegetables warm or at room temperature.

This Greek•style roasted vegetable dish is a delicious and diabetes•friendly side or main dish. The combination of roasted vegetables, feta, and herbs provides fiber, vitamins, and minerals without a lot of extra calories or carbs. Adjust the amount of feta to control the sodium content if needed.

38. Greek•Style Stuffed Peppers

Ingredient:

• 6 medium bell peppers (any color)
• 1 lb ground turkey or lean ground beef
• 1 cup cooked brown rice
• 1 small onion, finely chopped
• 2 cloves garlic, minced
• 1 tsp dried oregano
• 1/2 tsp dried basil
• 1/4 tsp salt
• 1/4 tsp black pepper
• 1 (14.5 oz) can diced tomatoes, drained
• 1/2 cup crumbled feta cheese

Instructions:

1. Preheat oven to 375°F. Cut the tops off the peppers and remove the seeds and membranes. Place the peppers in a baking dish.

2. In a large bowl, combine the ground turkey/beef, cooked rice, onion, garlic, oregano, basil, salt, and pepper. Mix well.

3. Stuff the pepper cavities evenly with the meat mixture. Top each stuffed pepper with some of the diced tomatoes.

4. Cover the baking dish with foil and bake for 40•45 minutes, until the peppers are tender and the filling is cooked through.

5. Remove the foil, sprinkle the feta cheese over the tops of the peppers, and bake for 5 more minutes.

6. Serve the stuffed peppers warm.

These Greek•style stuffed peppers are a delicious and diabetes•friendly meal. The lean protein, whole grains, and vegetables make it a nutritious option. Adjust the amount of feta cheese to control the sodium content if needed.

39. Greek•Style Green Beans with Tomatoes

Ingredient:

• 1 lb fresh green beans, trimmed
• 2 tbsp olive oil
• 1 onion, thinly sliced
• 3 cloves garlic, minced
• 1 (14.5 oz) can diced tomatoes, with juices
• 1 tsp dried oregano
• 1/4 tsp salt
• 1/4 tsp black pepper
• 2 tbsp crumbled feta cheese
• 2 tbsp chopped fresh parsley

Instructions:

1. Bring a large pot of salted water to a boil. Add the green beans and cook for 5•7 minutes, until tender•crisp. Drain and set aside.

2. In a large skillet, heat the olive oil over medium heat. Add the sliced onion and cook for 5 minutes, until softened.

3. Add the minced garlic and cook for 1 minute, until fragrant.

4. Pour in the can of diced tomatoes with their juices. Stir in the oregano, salt, and pepper.

5. Add the cooked green beans to the skillet and toss to coat with the tomato mixture. Cook for 5•7 minutes, until the beans are heated through.

6. Remove from heat and sprinkle the crumbled feta cheese and chopped parsley over the top.

7. Serve the Greek•style green beans warm.

This Greek•style green bean dish is a delicious and diabetes•friendly side. The combination of fresh green beans, tomatoes, feta, and herbs provides fiber, vitamins, and minerals without a lot of extra calories or carbs. Adjust the amount of feta to control the sodium content if needed.

40. Greek Lemon Chicken

Ingredient:

- 1 lb boneless, skinless chicken breasts
- 2 tbsp olive oil
- 2 tbsp lemon juice
- 2 tsp dried oregano
- 1 tsp garlic powder
- 1/2 tsp salt
- 1/4 tsp black pepper
- 1 lemon, sliced
- 2 tbsp chopped fresh parsley

Instructions:

1. Preheat oven to 400°F. Lightly grease a baking dish.

2. In a shallow bowl, whisk together the olive oil, lemon juice, oregano, garlic powder, salt, and pepper.

3. Add the chicken breasts to the marinade and turn to coat both sides. Cover and refrigerate for 30 minutes to 1 hour.

4. Arrange the marinated chicken breasts in the prepared baking dish. Arrange the lemon slices around the chicken.

5. Bake for 25•30 minutes, until the chicken is cooked through and reaches an internal temperature of 165°F.

6. Remove from oven and sprinkle the chopped parsley over the top.

7. Serve the Greek lemon chicken warm.

This Greek lemon chicken is a delicious and diabetes•friendly main dish. The lemon, oregano, and garlic provide lots of flavor without a lot of extra calories or carbs. Pair it with a side salad or roasted vegetables for a complete, healthy meal.

41. Greek•Style Artichokes

Ingredient:

• 4 medium artichokes
• 2 tbsp olive oil
• 2 cloves garlic, minced
• 1 tsp dried oregano
• 1/4 tsp salt
• 1/4 tsp black pepper
• 1/4 cup crumbled feta cheese
• 2 tbsp lemon juice
• 2 tbsp chopped fresh parsley

Instructions:

1. Trim the artichokes: Cut off the stem at the base, then use kitchen shears to snip off the thorny tips of the leaves.

2. In a large pot, bring 2•3 inches of water to a boil. Place the artichokes in the pot, cover, and steam for 25•30 minutes, until the leaves pull off easily.

3. Drain the artichokes and let cool slightly. Once cool enough to handle, use your fingers to gently pull the leaves apart.

4. In a small bowl, mix together the olive oil, garlic, oregano, salt, and pepper.

5. Brush the artichoke leaves and hearts with the garlic•herb oil mixture.

6. Sprinkle the feta cheese over the top of the artichokes.

7. Drizzle the lemon juice over the artichokes and garnish with the chopped parsley.

8. Serve the Greek•style artichokes warm or at room temperature.

These Greek•style artichokes make a delicious and diabetes•friendly appetizer or side dish. The artichokes provide fiber, while the feta, lemon, and herbs add lots of flavor without a lot of extra calories or carbs.

42. Greek Cauliflower Salad

Ingredient:

• 1 head of cauliflower, cut into small florets (about 4 cups)
• 1/2 cup diced cucumber
• 1/2 cup halved cherry tomatoes
• 1/4 cup pitted kalamata olives, halved
• 2 tbsp crumbled feta cheese
• 2 tbsp chopped fresh parsley
• 2 tbsp olive oil
• 1 tbsp lemon juice
• 1 tsp dried oregano
• 1/4 tsp salt
• 1/4 tsp black pepper

Instructions:

1. In a large bowl, combine the cauliflower florets, diced cucumber, cherry tomatoes, kalamata olives, feta cheese, and chopped parsley.

2. In a small bowl, whisk together the olive oil, lemon juice, oregano, salt, and pepper.

3. Pour the dressing over the cauliflower salad and toss gently to coat.

4. Cover and refrigerate for at least 30 minutes to allow the flavors to meld.

5. Serve the Greek cauliflower salad chilled or at room temperature.

Nutritional Information (per serving):
Calories: 120
Total Fat: 9g
Saturated Fat: 2g
Carbohydrates: 8g
Fiber: 3g
Protein: 4g

This Greek cauliflower salad is a refreshing and diabetes•friendly side dish or light meal. The combination of crisp cauliflower, fresh vegetables, tangy feta, and herbs provides fiber, vitamins, and minerals without a lot of extra calories or carbs. Adjust the amount of feta cheese to control the sodium content if needed.

43. Greek•Style Lamb Meatballs

Ingredient:

- 1 lb ground lamb
- 1/2 cup whole wheat breadcrumbs
- 1 egg, lightly beaten
- 2 tbsp chopped fresh parsley
- 2 tsp dried oregano
- 1 tsp garlic powder
- 1/2 tsp salt
- 1/4 tsp black pepper
- 2 tbsp olive oil
- 1 (14.5 oz) can diced tomatoes
- 2 tbsp lemon juice
- 1/4 cup crumbled feta cheese

Instructions:

1. In a large bowl, combine the ground lamb, breadcrumbs, egg, parsley, oregano, garlic powder, salt, and pepper. Mix well until fully incorporated.

2. Roll the mixture into 1•inch meatballs, making about 20•24 meatballs total.

3. In a large skillet, heat the olive oil over medium•high heat. Add the meatballs and cook for 5•6 minutes, turning occasionally, until browned on all sides.

4. Pour in the can of diced tomatoes with their juices. Bring the mixture to a simmer, then reduce heat and let the meatballs simmer for 10•12 minutes, until cooked through.

5. Remove from heat and stir in the lemon juice.

6. Transfer the Greek•style lamb meatballs to a serving dish and sprinkle the crumbled feta cheese over the top.

7. Serve warm, over a bed of roasted vegetables or cauliflower rice.

These Greek•style lamb meatballs are a delicious and diabetes•friendly option. The lean lamb, whole wheat breadcrumbs, and vegetables provide protein, fiber, and nutrients without a lot of extra carbs. Adjust the amount of feta cheese to control the sodium content if needed.

44. Greek•Style Roasted Eggplant

Ingredient:

• 1 large eggplant, cut into 1•inch cubes (about 4 cups)
• 2 tbsp olive oil
• 1 tsp dried oregano
• 1/2 tsp garlic powder
• 1/4 tsp salt
• 1/4 tsp black pepper
• 2 tbsp crumbled feta cheese
• 2 tbsp chopped fresh parsley
• 1 tbsp lemon juice

Instructions:

1. Preheat oven to 400°F. Line a large baking sheet with parchment paper.

2. In a large bowl, toss the cubed eggplant with the olive oil, oregano, garlic powder, salt, and pepper until evenly coated.

3. Spread the seasoned eggplant in a single layer on the prepared baking sheet.

4. Roast for 25•30 minutes, stirring halfway, until the eggplant is tender and lightly browned.

5. Transfer the roasted eggplant to a serving dish. Sprinkle the crumbled feta cheese and chopped parsley over the top.

6. Drizzle the lemon juice over the eggplant.

7. Serve the Greek•style roasted eggplant warm or at room temperature.

This Greek•style roasted eggplant dish is a delicious and diabetes•friendly side or main dish. The combination of roasted eggplant, feta, herbs, and lemon provides fiber, vitamins, and minerals without a lot of extra calories or carbs. Adjust the amount of feta cheese to control the sodium content if needed.

45. Greek Chicken with Olives and Tomatoes

Ingredient:

- 1 lb boneless, skinless chicken breasts, cut into 1•inch pieces
- 2 tbsp olive oil
- 1 onion, diced
- 3 cloves garlic, minced
- 1 tsp dried oregano
- 1/2 tsp dried thyme
- 1/4 tsp salt
- 1/4 tsp black pepper
- 1 (14.5 oz) can diced tomatoes
- 1/2 cup pitted kalamata olives, halved
- 2 tbsp lemon juice
- 2 tbsp chopped fresh parsley

Instructions:

1. In a large skillet, heat the olive oil over medium•high heat. Add the chicken pieces and cook for 5•6 minutes, until lightly browned on all sides. Remove chicken from skillet and set aside.

2. Add the diced onion to the skillet and cook for 3•4 minutes, until softened. Add the minced garlic and cook for 1 minute more.

3. Stir in the oregano, thyme, salt, and pepper. Cook for 1 minute to toast the spices.

4. Pour in the can of diced tomatoes with their juices. Add the cooked chicken back to the skillet along with the halved kalamata olives.

5. Bring the mixture to a simmer and cook for 10•12 minutes, until the chicken is cooked through and the sauce has thickened slightly.

6. Remove from heat and stir in the lemon juice and chopped parsley.

7. Serve the Greek chicken with olives and tomatoes warm, over a bed of steamed vegetables or cauliflower rice.

This Greek•style chicken dish is a delicious and diabetes•friendly meal. The lean chicken, tomatoes, olives, and herbs provide protein, fiber, and nutrients without a lot of extra carbs or calories. Adjust the amount of olives to control the sodium content if needed.

46. Greek•Style Broccoli

Ingredient:

• 1 lb broccoli florets
• 2 tbsp olive oil
• 2 cloves garlic, minced
• 1 tsp dried oregano
• 1/4 tsp salt
• 1/4 tsp black pepper
• 2 tbsp crumbled feta cheese
• 1 tbsp lemon juice
• 2 tbsp chopped fresh parsley

Instructions:

1. Bring a large pot of salted water to a boil. Add the broccoli florets and cook for 3•4 minutes, until tender•crisp. Drain and set aside.

2. In a large skillet, heat the olive oil over medium heat. Add the minced garlic and cook for 1 minute, until fragrant.

3. Add the cooked broccoli florets to the skillet. Sprinkle with the dried oregano, salt, and pepper. Toss to coat the broccoli.

4. Cook for 2•3 minutes, stirring occasionally, until the broccoli is heated through.

5. Remove from heat and transfer the Greek•style broccoli to a serving dish.

6. Sprinkle the crumbled feta cheese and chopped parsley over the top. Drizzle with the lemon juice. Serve the broccoli warm.

Nutritional Information (per serving):
Calories: 100
Total Fat: 7g
Saturated Fat: 2g
Carbohydrates: 7g
Fiber: 3g
Protein: 4g

This Greek•style broccoli dish is a delicious and diabetes•friendly side. The combination of tender•crisp broccoli, feta, lemon, and herbs provides fiber, vitamins, and minerals without a lot of extra calories or carbs. Adjust the amount of feta cheese to control the sodium content if needed.

47. Greek•Style Brussels Sprouts

Ingredient:

- 1 lb Brussels sprouts, trimmed and halved
- 2 tbsp olive oil
- 1 tsp dried oregano
- 1/2 tsp garlic powder
- 1/4 tsp salt
- 1/4 tsp black pepper
- 2 tbsp crumbled feta cheese
- 1 tbsp lemon juice
- 2 tbsp chopped fresh parsley

Instructions:

1. Preheat oven to 400°F. Line a large baking sheet with parchment paper.

2. In a large bowl, toss the Brussels sprouts with the olive oil, oregano, garlic powder, salt, and pepper until evenly coated.

3. Spread the seasoned Brussels sprouts in a single layer on the prepared baking sheet.

4. Roast for 20•25 minutes, stirring halfway, until the Brussels sprouts are tender and lightly browned.

5. Transfer the roasted Brussels sprouts to a serving dish. Sprinkle the crumbled feta cheese and chopped parsley over the top.

6. Drizzle the lemon juice over the Brussels sprouts. Serve the Greek•style Brussels sprouts warm.

Nutritional Information (per serving):
Calories: 110
Total Fat: 7g
Saturated Fat: 2g
Carbohydrates: 9g
Fiber: 4g
Protein: 4g

These Greek•style Brussels sprouts make a delicious and diabetes•friendly side dish. The roasted Brussels sprouts, feta, lemon, and herbs provide fiber, vitamins, and minerals without a lot of extra calories or carbs. Adjust the amount of feta cheese to control the sodium content if needed.

48. Greek•Style Cucumber Salad

Ingredient:

• 2 medium cucumbers, sliced
• 1/2 red onion, thinly sliced
• 1/2 cup halved cherry tomatoes
• 1/4 cup pitted kalamata olives, halved
• 2 tbsp crumbled feta cheese
• 2 tbsp chopped fresh dill
• 2 tbsp olive oil
• 1 tbsp red wine vinegar
• 1 tsp dried oregano
• 1/4 tsp salt
• 1/4 tsp black pepper

Instructions:

1. In a large bowl, combine the sliced cucumbers, red onion, cherry tomatoes, and kalamata olives.

2. In a small bowl, whisk together the olive oil, red wine vinegar, oregano, salt, and pepper.

3. Pour the dressing over the cucumber salad and toss gently to coat.

4. Sprinkle the crumbled feta cheese and chopped fresh dill over the top.

5. Cover and refrigerate for at least 30 minutes to allow the flavors to meld. Serve the Greek•style cucumber salad chilled.

Nutritional Information (per serving):
Calories: 100
Total Fat: 7g
Saturated Fat: 2g
Carbohydrates: 8g
Fiber: 2g
Protein: 2g

This refreshing Greek•style cucumber salad is a perfect diabetes•friendly side dish or light meal. The combination of crisp cucumbers, tangy feta, and fresh herbs provides fiber, vitamins, and minerals without a lot of extra calories or carbs. Adjust the amount of feta cheese to control the sodium content if needed.

49. Greek•Style Roasted Potatoes

Ingredient:

• 2 lbs Yukon Gold potatoes, cut into 1•inch cubes
• 2 tbsp olive oil
• 1 tsp dried oregano
• 1 tsp garlic powder
• 1/2 tsp salt
• 1/4 tsp black pepper
• 2 tbsp lemon juice
• 2 tbsp chopped fresh parsley
• 2 tbsp crumbled feta cheese

Instructions:

1. Preheat oven to 400°F. Line a large baking sheet with parchment paper.

2. In a large bowl, toss the cubed potatoes with the olive oil, oregano, garlic powder, salt, and pepper until evenly coated.

3. Spread the seasoned potato cubes in a single layer on the prepared baking sheet.

4. Roast for 30•35 minutes, flipping halfway, until the potatoes are tender and lightly browned.

5. Remove the potatoes from the oven and drizzle with the lemon juice. Toss to coat.

6. Transfer the roasted potatoes to a serving dish and sprinkle with the chopped parsley and crumbled feta cheese. Serve the Greek•style roasted potatoes warm.

Nutritional Information (per serving):
Calories: 180
Total Fat: 7g
Saturated Fat: 2g
Carbohydrates: 24g
Fiber: 3g
Protein: 4g

These Greek•style roasted potatoes are a delicious and diabetes•friendly side dish. The combination of roasted potatoes, lemon, herbs, and feta provides lots of flavor without a lot of extra calories or carbs. Adjust the amount of feta cheese to control the sodium content if needed.

50. Greek•Style Stuffed Tomatoes

Ingredient:

• 6 medium tomatoes
• 1/2 cup cooked quinoa
• 1/4 cup crumbled feta cheese
• 2 tbsp chopped fresh parsley
• 1 tbsp olive oil
• 1 tsp dried oregano
• 1/4 tsp salt
• 1/4 tsp black pepper

Instructions:

1. Preheat oven to 375°F. Slice the tops off the tomatoes and scoop out the seeds and pulp, leaving a hollow shell. Finely chop the scooped out tomato flesh.

2. In a medium bowl, combine the chopped tomato flesh, cooked quinoa, feta cheese, parsley, olive oil, oregano, salt, and pepper. Mix well.

3. Stuff the tomato shells evenly with the quinoa•feta mixture.

4. Place the stuffed tomatoes in a baking dish.

5. Bake for 20•25 minutes, until the tomatoes are tender and the filling is heated through.

6. Serve the Greek•style stuffed tomatoes warm.

Nutritional Information (per serving):
Calories: 100
Total Fat: 5g
Saturated Fat: 2g
Carbohydrates: 10g
Fiber: 2g
Protein: 4g

These Greek•style stuffed tomatoes make a delicious and diabetes•friendly appetizer or side dish. The combination of fresh tomatoes, quinoa, feta, and herbs provides fiber, protein, and nutrients without a lot of extra calories or carbs. Adjust the amount of feta cheese to control the sodium content if needed.

51. Greek•Style Grilled Vegetables

Ingredient:

- 1 zucchini, sliced into 1/2•inch thick rounds
- 1 yellow squash, sliced into 1/2•inch thick rounds
- 1 red bell pepper, cut into 1•inch pieces
- 1 red onion, cut into 1•inch wedges
- 2 tbsp olive oil
- 1 tsp dried oregano
- 1/2 tsp garlic powder
- 1/4 tsp salt
- 1/4 tsp black pepper
- 2 tbsp crumbled feta cheese
- 1 tbsp chopped fresh parsley
- 1 tbsp lemon juice

Instructions:

1. Preheat grill or grill pan to medium•high heat.

2. In a large bowl, toss the zucchini, yellow squash, bell pepper, and onion with the olive oil, oregano, garlic powder, salt, and pepper until evenly coated.

3. Grill the vegetables for 8•10 minutes, turning occasionally, until tender and lightly charred.

4. Transfer the grilled vegetables to a serving dish. Sprinkle the crumbled feta cheese and chopped parsley over the top.

5. Drizzle the lemon juice over the vegetables. Serve the Greek•style grilled vegetables warm.

Nutritional Information (per serving):
Calories: 120
Total Fat: 8g
Saturated Fat: 2g

This Greek•style grilled vegetable dish is a delicious and diabetes•friendly side or main dish. The combination of grilled vegetables, feta, and herbs provides fiber, vitamins, and minerals without a lot of extra calories or carbs. Adjust the amount of feta cheese to control the sodium content if needed.

52. Greek•Style Lemon Potatoes

Ingredient:

• 2 lbs Yukon Gold potatoes, cut into 1•inch cubes
• 2 tbsp olive oil
• 2 tbsp lemon juice
• 1 tsp dried oregano
• 1 tsp garlic powder
• 1/2 tsp salt
• 1/4 tsp black pepper
• 2 tbsp chopped fresh parsley
• 2 tbsp crumbled feta cheese

Instructions:

1. Preheat oven to 400°F. Line a large baking sheet with parchment paper.

2. In a large bowl, toss the cubed potatoes with the olive oil, lemon juice, oregano, garlic powder, salt, and pepper until evenly coated.

3. Spread the seasoned potato cubes in a single layer on the prepared baking sheet.

4. Roast for 30•35 minutes, flipping halfway, until the potatoes are tender and lightly browned.

5. Transfer the roasted Greek•style lemon potatoes to a serving dish.

6. Sprinkle the chopped parsley and crumbled feta cheese over the top.

7. Serve the potatoes warm.

Nutritional Information (per serving):
Calories: 180
Total Fat: 7g

These Greek•style lemon potatoes are a delicious and diabetes•friendly side dish. The combination of roasted potatoes, lemon, herbs, and feta provides lots of flavor without a lot of extra calories or carbs. Adjust the amount of feta cheese to control the sodium content if needed.

53. Greek•Style Stuffed Mushrooms

Ingredient:

• 12 large mushrooms, stems removed and finely chopped
• 2 tbsp olive oil
• 1/4 cup diced onion
• 2 cloves garlic, minced
• 1/4 cup crumbled feta cheese
• 2 tbsp chopped fresh parsley
• 1 tsp dried oregano
• 1/4 tsp salt
• 1/4 tsp black pepper

Instructions:

1. Preheat oven to 375°F. Lightly grease a baking sheet.

2. In a skillet, heat the olive oil over medium heat. Add the chopped mushroom stems, diced onion, and minced garlic. Cook for 3•4 minutes, until the vegetables are softened.

3. Remove the skillet from heat and stir in the crumbled feta cheese, chopped parsley, dried oregano, salt, and pepper.

4. Stuff the mushroom caps evenly with the feta•herb filling.

5. Arrange the stuffed mushrooms on the prepared baking sheet.

6. Bake for 12•15 minutes, until the mushrooms are tender and the filling is heated through. Serve the Greek•style stuffed mushrooms warm.

Nutritional Information (per serving):
Calories: 50
Total Fat: 4g
Saturated Fat: 1g
Carbohydrates: 3g
Fiber: 1g

These Greek•style stuffed mushrooms make a delicious and diabetes•friendly appetizer or snack. The combination of savory mushrooms, tangy feta, and fresh herbs provides flavor without a lot of extra calories or carbs. Adjust the amount of feta cheese to control the sodium content if needed.

54. Greek•Style Steamed Mussels

Ingredient:

• 2 lbs mussels, scrubbed and debearded
• 2 tbsp olive oil
• 3 cloves garlic, minced
• 1 cup diced tomatoes
• 1/2 cup dry white wine
• 1 tsp dried oregano
• 1/4 tsp salt
• 1/4 tsp black pepper
• 2 tbsp chopped fresh parsley
• 2 tbsp crumbled feta cheese

Instructions:

1. In a large pot or Dutch oven, heat the olive oil over medium heat. Add the minced garlic and cook for 1 minute, until fragrant.

2. Add the diced tomatoes, white wine, oregano, salt, and pepper. Bring the mixture to a simmer.

3. Add the mussels to the pot, cover, and steam for 5•7 minutes, until the mussels have opened up.

4. Discard any mussels that did not open.

5. Transfer the steamed mussels to a serving bowl. Pour the tomato•wine broth over the top.

6. Sprinkle the chopped parsley and crumbled feta cheese over the mussels. Serve the Greek•style steamed mussels immediately, with crusty bread for dipping if desired.

Nutritional Information (per serving):
Calories: 220
Total Fat: 9g

These Greek•style steamed mussels make a delicious and diabetes•friendly seafood dish. The mussels provide lean protein, while the tomatoes, wine, and feta add lots of flavor without a lot of extra carbs or calories. Adjust the amount of feta cheese to control the sodium content if needed.

55. Greek•Style Lemon Garlic Shrimp

Ingredient:

• 1 lb large shrimp, peeled and deveined
• 2 tbsp olive oil
• 3 cloves garlic, minced
• 1 tsp dried oregano
• 1/4 tsp red pepper flakes (optional)
• 1/4 tsp salt
• 1/4 tsp black pepper
• 2 tbsp lemon juice
• 2 tbsp chopped fresh parsley
• 2 tbsp crumbled feta cheese

Instructions:

1. In a large skillet, heat the olive oil over medium•high heat.

2. Add the minced garlic and cook for 1 minute, until fragrant.

3. Add the shrimp, oregano, red pepper flakes (if using), salt, and pepper. Toss to coat the shrimp.

4. Cook the shrimp for 3•4 minutes per side, until they are opaque and cooked through.

5. Remove the skillet from heat and stir in the lemon juice and chopped parsley.

6. Transfer the Greek•style lemon garlic shrimp to a serving dish and sprinkle the crumbled feta cheese over the top. Serve the shrimp warm, with lemon wedges if desired.

Nutritional Information (per serving):
Calories: 180
Total Fat: 9g
Saturated Fat: 2g
Carbohydrates: 3g

This Greek•style lemon garlic shrimp is a delicious and diabetes•friendly seafood dish. The shrimp provides lean protein, while the lemon, garlic, and feta add lots of flavor without a lot of extra carbs or calories. Adjust the amount of feta cheese to control the sodium content if needed.

56. Greek•Style Baked Tofu

Ingredient:

• 1 block (14 oz) extra•firm tofu, pressed and cut into 1•inch cubes
• 2 tbsp olive oil
• 2 tbsp lemon juice
• 1 tsp dried oregano
• 1/2 tsp garlic powder
• 1/4 tsp salt
• 1/4 tsp black pepper
• 2 tbsp crumbled feta cheese
• 2 tbsp chopped fresh parsley

Instructions:

1. Preheat oven to 400°F. Line a baking sheet with parchment paper.

2. In a large bowl, toss the tofu cubes with the olive oil, lemon juice, oregano, garlic powder, salt, and pepper until evenly coated.

3. Arrange the seasoned tofu cubes in a single layer on the prepared baking sheet.

4. Bake for 20•25 minutes, flipping halfway, until the tofu is lightly browned and crispy.

5. Transfer the baked Greek•style tofu to a serving dish. Sprinkle the crumbled feta cheese and chopped parsley over the top. Serve the tofu warm.

Nutritional Information (per serving):
Calories: 150
Total Fat: 10g
Saturated Fat: 2g
Carbohydrates: 5g
Fiber: 2g
Protein: 12g

This Greek•style baked tofu is a delicious and diabetes•friendly protein option. The combination of crispy tofu, tangy feta, and fresh herbs provides flavor and nutrients without a lot of extra carbs or calories. Adjust the amount of feta cheese to control the sodium content if needed.

57. Greek•Style Spaghetti Squash

Ingredient:

• 1 medium spaghetti squash, halved lengthwise and seeded
• 2 tbsp olive oil
• 1 clove garlic, minced
• 1 tsp dried oregano
• 1/4 tsp salt
• 1/4 tsp black pepper
• 1/2 cup diced tomatoes
• 2 tbsp crumbled feta cheese
• 2 tbsp chopped fresh parsley

Instructions:

1. Preheat oven to 400°F. Place the spaghetti squash halves cut•side down on a baking sheet. Bake for 30•40 minutes, until tender when pierced with a fork.

2. Remove the spaghetti squash from the oven and let cool slightly. Use a fork to scrape the flesh into strands.

3. In a large skillet, heat the olive oil over medium heat. Add the minced garlic and cook for 1 minute, until fragrant.

4. Add the spaghetti squash strands, oregano, salt, and pepper. Toss to coat the squash.

5. Stir in the diced tomatoes and cook for 2•3 minutes, until heated through.

6. Remove from heat and transfer the Greek•style spaghetti squash to a serving dish.

7. Sprinkle the crumbled feta cheese and chopped parsley over the top. Serve warm.

Nutritional Information (per serving):
Calories: 120
Total Fat: 7g

This Greek•style spaghetti squash is a delicious and diabetes•friendly alternative to traditional pasta. The combination of roasted squash, tomatoes, feta, and herbs provides fiber, vitamins, and minerals without a lot of extra carbs. Adjust the amount of feta cheese to control the sodium content if needed.

58. Greek•Style Tuna Salad

Ingredient:

• 2 (5 oz) cans tuna, drained
• 1/4 cup plain Greek yogurt
• 2 tbsp diced cucumber
• 2 tbsp diced tomatoes
• 2 tbsp crumbled feta cheese
• 1 tbsp chopped fresh parsley
• 1 tsp lemon juice
• 1/4 tsp dried oregano
• 1/4 tsp salt
• 1/4 tsp black pepper

Instructions:

1. In a medium bowl, combine the drained tuna, Greek yogurt, diced cucumber, diced tomatoes, crumbled feta cheese, chopped parsley, lemon juice, dried oregano, salt, and pepper. Mix well.

2. Taste and adjust seasonings as needed.

3. Serve the Greek•style tuna salad chilled, on a bed of mixed greens, or with whole grain crackers or pita bread.

Nutritional Information (per serving):
Calories: 150
Total Fat: 6g
Saturated Fat: 2g
Carbohydrates: 4g
Fiber: 1g
Protein: 20g

This Greek•style tuna salad is a delicious and diabetes•friendly option for a light meal or snack. The combination of tuna, Greek yogurt, vegetables, and herbs provides protein, fiber, and nutrients without a lot of extra carbs or calories. Adjust the amount of feta cheese to control the sodium content if needed.

59. Greek•Style Scrambled Eggs

Ingredient:

- 6 large eggs
- 2 tbsp milk
- 1 tsp olive oil
- 2 tbsp diced onion
- 1 clove garlic, minced
- 1 tsp dried oregano
- 1/4 tsp salt
- 1/4 tsp black pepper
- 2 tbsp crumbled feta cheese
- 2 tbsp chopped fresh parsley

Instructions:

1. In a medium bowl, whisk together the eggs and milk until well combined.

2. In a nonstick skillet, heat the olive oil over medium heat. Add the diced onion and cook for 2•3 minutes, until softened.

3. Add the minced garlic and cook for 1 minute, until fragrant.

4. Pour the egg mixture into the skillet. Sprinkle the dried oregano, salt, and pepper over the top.

5. Use a spatula to gently stir and scramble the eggs, cooking for 2•3 minutes until they are softly scrambled.

6. Remove the skillet from heat and stir in the crumbled feta cheese.

7. Transfer the Greek•style scrambled eggs to a plate and garnish with the chopped fresh parsley. Serve the scrambled eggs warm.

These Greek•style scrambled eggs are a delicious and diabetes•friendly breakfast option. The combination of eggs, feta, and herbs provides protein, vitamins, and minerals without a lot of extra carbs. Adjust the amount of feta cheese to control the sodium content if needed.

60. Greek•Style Baked Beans

Ingredient:

• 2 (15 oz) cans white beans, drained and rinsed
• 1 (15 oz) can diced tomatoes
• 1 onion, diced
• 3 cloves garlic, minced
• 1 tablespoon olive oil
• 1 teaspoon dried oregano
• 1/2 teaspoon ground cinnamon
• 1/4 teaspoon ground cloves
• 1/4 teaspoon salt
• 1/4 teaspoon black pepper
• 1/4 cup crumbled feta cheese

Instructions:

1. Preheat your oven to 375°F (190°C).

2. In a large oven•safe skillet or baking dish, combine the drained and rinsed white beans, diced tomatoes, diced onion, and minced garlic. Drizzle with the olive oil and stir to coat.

3. Add the dried oregano, ground cinnamon, ground cloves, salt, and black pepper. Stir to combine.

4. Bake the beans in the preheated oven for 30•35 minutes, or until the beans are heated through and the flavors have melded.

5. Remove the beans from the oven and sprinkle the crumbled feta cheese on top.

6. Serve the Greek•Style Baked Beans warm, either as a side dish or as a main course with a side salad.

This dish is high in fiber and protein from the beans, and the feta cheese provides a tangy, creamy contrast. The cinnamon and cloves add a warm, aromatic flavor that complements the other Mediterranean•inspired ingredients.

61. Greek·Style Cabbage Salad

Ingredient:

• 1 head green cabbage, shredded (about 6 cups)
• 1 cup cherry tomatoes, halved
• 1/2 cup crumbled feta cheese
• 1/4 cup sliced black olives
• 1/4 cup thinly sliced red onion
• 2 tablespoons red wine vinegar
• 1 tablespoon olive oil
• 1 tablespoon lemon juice
• 1 teaspoon dried oregano
• 1/4 teaspoon salt
• 1/4 teaspoon black pepper

Instructions:

1. In a large bowl, combine the shredded cabbage, cherry tomatoes, feta cheese, black olives, and red onion.

2. In a small bowl, whisk together the red wine vinegar, olive oil, lemon juice, oregano, salt, and black pepper.

3. Pour the dressing over the cabbage mixture and toss gently to coat.

4. Refrigerate for at least 30 minutes to allow the flavors to blend.

5. Serve chilled or at room temperature.

This salad is low in carbs and high in fiber, making it a great option for people with diabetes. The feta cheese and olives provide healthy fats, while the cabbage and tomatoes are packed with vitamins and antioxidants.

62. Greek•Style Salmon Fillets

Ingredient:

- 4 (6 oz) salmon fillets
- 2 tablespoons olive oil
- 2 tablespoons lemon juice
- 2 cloves garlic, minced
- 1 teaspoon dried oregano
- 1/2 teaspoon salt
- 1/4 teaspoon black pepper
- 1/4 cup crumbled feta cheese
- 2 tablespoons chopped fresh parsley

Instructions:

1. Preheat your oven to 400°F (200°C).

2. In a small bowl, whisk together the olive oil, lemon juice, minced garlic, dried oregano, salt, and black pepper.

3. Place the salmon fillets in a baking dish or on a parchment•lined baking sheet.

4. Drizzle the olive oil and lemon juice mixture over the salmon fillets, making sure to coat them evenly.

5. Bake the salmon in the preheated oven for 12•15 minutes, or until the fish flakes easily with a fork.

6. Remove the salmon from the oven and sprinkle the crumbled feta cheese and chopped fresh parsley over the top.

7. Serve the Greek•Style Salmon Fillets immediately, while hot.

This dish is high in protein from the salmon, and the feta cheese provides a tangy, creamy contrast. The lemon, garlic, and oregano flavors complement the salmon beautifully, making this a delicious and healthy option for people with diabetes.

63. Greek•Style Kale Salad

Ingredient:

• 6 cups chopped kale, stems removed
• 1/2 cup diced cucumber
• 1/2 cup halved cherry tomatoes
• 1/4 cup pitted kalamata olives, halved
• 2 tbsp crumbled feta cheese
• 2 tbsp chopped fresh parsley
• 2 tbsp olive oil
• 1 tbsp red wine vinegar
• 1 tsp Dijon mustard
• 1 tsp dried oregano
• 1/4 tsp salt
• 1/4 tsp black pepper

Instructions:

1. In a large bowl, combine the chopped kale, diced cucumber, cherry tomatoes, and kalamata olives.

2. In a small bowl, whisk together the olive oil, red wine vinegar, Dijon mustard, dried oregano, salt, and pepper.

3. Pour the dressing over the kale salad and toss to coat. Sprinkle the crumbled feta cheese and chopped parsley over the top.

4. Cover and refrigerate for at least 30 minutes to allow the flavors to meld. Serve the Greek•style kale salad chilled.

Nutritional Information (per serving):
Calories: 130
Total Fat: 9g
Saturated Fat: 2g
Carbohydrates: 9g
Fiber: 2g
Protein: 4g

This Greek•style kale salad is a delicious and diabetes•friendly option. The combination of nutrient•dense kale, fresh vegetables, tangy feta, and herbs provides fiber, vitamins, and minerals without a lot of extra calories or carbs. Adjust the amount of feta cheese to control the sodium content if needed.

64. Greek•Style Cucumber Soup

Ingredient:

• 2 cups diced cucumber
• 1 cup plain Greek yogurt
• 1/4 cup low•sodium vegetable broth
• 2 tbsp lemon juice
• 1 clove garlic, minced
• 1 tsp dried dill
• 1/4 tsp salt
• 1/4 tsp black pepper
• 2 tbsp crumbled feta cheese
• 1 tbsp chopped fresh parsley

Instructions:

1. In a blender or food processor, combine the diced cucumber, Greek yogurt, vegetable broth, lemon juice, minced garlic, dried dill, salt, and pepper. Blend until smooth.

2. Transfer the cucumber soup to a serving bowl and refrigerate for at least 30 minutes to allow the flavors to meld.

3. When ready to serve, ladle the chilled Greek•style cucumber soup into bowls.

4. Sprinkle the crumbled feta cheese and chopped parsley over the top of each serving.

Nutritional Information (per serving):
Calories: 90
Total Fat: 4g
Saturated Fat: 2g
Carbohydrates: 8g
Fiber: 1g
Protein: 6g

This refreshing Greek•style cucumber soup is a delicious and diabetes•friendly option. The combination of cool cucumbers, tangy Greek yogurt, and fresh herbs provides fiber, protein, and nutrients without a lot of extra calories or carbs. Adjust the amount of feta cheese to control the sodium content if needed.

65. Greek•Style Baked Acorn Squash

Ingredient:

- 1 medium acorn squash, halved and seeded
- 2 tbsp olive oil
- 1 tsp dried oregano
- 1/2 tsp garlic powder
- 1/4 tsp salt
- 1/4 tsp black pepper
- 2 tbsp crumbled feta cheese
- 2 tbsp chopped fresh parsley

Instructions:

1. Preheat oven to 400°F. Line a baking sheet with parchment paper.

2. Place the acorn squash halves cut•side up on the prepared baking sheet.

3. In a small bowl, mix together the olive oil, dried oregano, garlic powder, salt, and pepper.

4. Brush the seasoned oil mixture over the cut surfaces of the acorn squash.

5. Roast for 30•40 minutes, until the squash is tender when pierced with a fork.

6. Remove the baked acorn squash from the oven and transfer the halves to a serving dish.

7. Sprinkle the crumbled feta cheese and chopped parsley over the top of the squash. Serve the Greek•style baked acorn squash warm.

Nutritional Information (per serving):
Calories: 150
Total Fat: 8g
Saturated Fat: 2g
Carbohydrates: 18g

This Greek•style baked acorn squash is a delicious and diabetes•friendly side dish. The roasted squash, feta, and herbs provide fiber, vitamins, and minerals without a lot of extra calories or carbs. Adjust the amount of feta cheese to control the sodium content if needed.

66. Greek•Style Spinach Salad

Ingredient:

- 6 cups baby spinach leaves
- 1/2 cup diced cucumber
- 1/2 cup halved cherry tomatoes
- 1/4 cup pitted kalamata olives, halved
- 2 tbsp crumbled feta cheese
- 2 tbsp chopped fresh dill
- 2 tbsp olive oil
- 1 tbsp red wine vinegar
- 1 tsp Dijon mustard
- 1 tsp dried oregano
- 1/4 tsp salt
- 1/4 tsp black pepper

Instructions:

1. In a large bowl, combine the baby spinach leaves, diced cucumber, cherry tomatoes, and kalamata olives.

2. In a small bowl, whisk together the olive oil, red wine vinegar, Dijon mustard, dried oregano, salt, and pepper.

3. Pour the dressing over the spinach salad and toss to coat. Sprinkle the crumbled feta cheese and chopped fresh dill over the top. Serve the Greek•style spinach salad immediately.

Nutritional Information (per serving):
Calories: 120
Total Fat: 9g
Saturated Fat: 2g
Carbohydrates: 7g
Fiber: 2g
Protein: 4g

This Greek•style spinach salad is a delicious and diabetes•friendly option. The combination of nutrient•dense spinach, fresh vegetables, tangy feta, and herbs provides fiber, vitamins, and minerals without a lot of extra calories or carbs. Adjust the amount of feta cheese to control the sodium content if needed.

67. Greek•Style Cauliflower Mash

Ingredient:

- 1 large head of cauliflower, cut into florets
- 2 tablespoons olive oil
- 2 cloves garlic, minced
- 1/4 cup crumbled feta cheese
- 2 tablespoons lemon juice
- 1 teaspoon dried oregano
- 1/4 teaspoon salt
- 1/4 teaspoon black pepper

Instructions:

1. In a large pot, bring a few inches of water to a boil. Add the cauliflower florets, cover, and steam for 10•12 minutes, or until the cauliflower is very tender.

2. Drain the cauliflower and transfer it to a food processor or high•powered blender.

3. Add the olive oil, minced garlic, crumbled feta cheese, lemon juice, dried oregano, salt, and black pepper to the food processor or blender.

4. Blend or process the mixture until it reaches a smooth, creamy consistency, scraping down the sides as needed.

5. Taste and adjust seasoning as needed, adding more salt, pepper, or lemon juice to your preference.

6. Transfer the Greek•Style Cauliflower Mash to a serving bowl and serve warm.

This cauliflower mash is a great low•carb alternative to traditional mashed potatoes. The feta cheese, lemon, and oregano give it a delicious Greek•inspired flavor. It's a perfect side dish for people with diabetes, as it's high in fiber and low in carbs.

68. Greek•Style Pork Tenderloin

Ingredient:

- 1 lb pork tenderloin
- 2 tbsp olive oil
- 2 tbsp lemon juice
- 1 tsp dried oregano
- 1 tsp garlic powder
- 1/2 tsp salt
- 1/4 tsp black pepper
- 2 tbsp crumbled feta cheese
- 2 tbsp chopped fresh parsley

Instructions:

1. In a shallow dish, combine the olive oil, lemon juice, oregano, garlic powder, salt, and pepper. Add the pork tenderloin and turn to coat both sides with the marinade. Cover and refrigerate for 30 minutes to 1 hour.

2. Preheat oven to 400°F. Line a baking sheet with parchment paper.

3. Place the marinated pork tenderloin on the prepared baking sheet.

4. Roast for 20•25 minutes, until the internal temperature reaches 145°F.

5. Remove the pork from the oven and let rest for 5 minutes.

6. Slice the pork tenderloin and transfer to a serving dish. Sprinkle the crumbled feta cheese and chopped parsley over the top. Serve the Greek•style pork tenderloin warm.

Nutritional Information (per serving):
Calories: 220
Total Fat: 10g
Saturated Fat: 3g
Carbohydrates: 2g
Fiber: 0g
Protein: 28g

This Greek•style pork tenderloin is a delicious and diabetes•friendly main dish. The lean pork, lemon, oregano, and feta provide lots of flavor without a lot of extra calories or carbs. Adjust the amount of feta cheese to control the sodium content if needed.

69. Greek•Style Steamed Broccoli

Ingredient:

• 1 lb broccoli florets
• 2 tablespoons olive oil
• 2 cloves garlic, minced
• 2 tablespoons lemon juice
• 2 tablespoons crumbled feta cheese
• 1 teaspoon dried oregano
• 1/4 teaspoon salt
• 1/4 teaspoon black pepper

Instructions:

1. In a steamer basket or saucepan with a small amount of water, steam the broccoli florets for 5•7 minutes, or until tender but still crisp.

2. Drain the broccoli and transfer it to a serving bowl.

3. In a small bowl, whisk together the olive oil, minced garlic, lemon juice, crumbled feta cheese, dried oregano, salt, and black pepper.

4. Pour the dressing over the steamed broccoli and toss gently to coat.

5. Serve the Greek•Style Steamed Broccoli warm or at room temperature.

This dish is a simple and flavorful way to enjoy broccoli. The lemon, garlic, and oregano provide a Mediterranean•inspired flavor, while the feta cheese adds a creamy, tangy element. It's a great side dish that's low in carbs and high in fiber, making it a suitable option for people with diabetes.

70. Greek•Style Beef Kabobs

Ingredient:

• 1 lb beef sirloin or tenderloin, cut into 1•inch cubes
• 1 red onion, cut into 1•inch pieces
• 1 red bell pepper, cut into 1•inch pieces
• 1 yellow bell pepper, cut into 1•inch pieces
• 8 cherry tomatoes
• 2 tablespoons olive oil
• 2 tablespoons lemon juice
• 2 cloves garlic, minced
• 1 teaspoon dried oregano
• 1/2 teaspoon salt
• 1/4 teaspoon black pepper
• 2 tablespoons crumbled feta cheese

Instructions:

1. In a large bowl, combine the beef cubes, onion, red bell pepper, yellow bell pepper, and cherry tomatoes.

2. In a small bowl, whisk together the olive oil, lemon juice, minced garlic, dried oregano, salt, and black pepper.

3. Pour the marinade over the beef and vegetable mixture and toss to coat everything evenly.

4. Thread the marinated beef and vegetables onto skewers, alternating the ingredients.

5. Preheat your grill or grill pan to medium•high heat.

6. Grill the kabobs for 8•10 minutes, turning occasionally, until the beef is cooked through and the vegetables are tender.

7. Transfer the grilled kabobs to a serving platter and sprinkle the crumbled feta cheese over the top. Serve the Greek•Style Beef Kabobs immediately.

This dish is a great source of protein from the beef, and the vegetables provide fiber and important vitamins and minerals. The feta cheese adds a tangy, creamy element to the kabobs. It's a delicious and healthy option for people with diabetes.

71. Greek•Style Quinoa Salad

Ingredient:

- 1 cup uncooked quinoa, rinsed
- 2 cups low•sodium vegetable or chicken broth
- 1 cup cherry tomatoes, halved
- 1 cucumber, diced
- 1/2 cup crumbled feta cheese
- 1/4 cup sliced kalamata olives
- 1/4 cup thinly sliced red onion
- 2 tablespoons chopped fresh parsley
- 2 tablespoons lemon juice
- 1 tablespoon olive oil
- 1 teaspoon dried oregano
- 1/4 teaspoon salt
- 1/4 teaspoon black pepper

Instructions:

1. In a medium saucepan, combine the rinsed quinoa and broth. Bring to a boil, then reduce heat to low, cover, and simmer for 15•20 minutes, or until the quinoa is tender and the liquid is absorbed.

2. Transfer the cooked quinoa to a large bowl and let it cool slightly.

3. Add the cherry tomatoes, diced cucumber, crumbled feta cheese, sliced kalamata olives, thinly sliced red onion, and chopped fresh parsley to the bowl with the quinoa.

4. In a small bowl, whisk together the lemon juice, olive oil, dried oregano, salt, and black pepper.

5. Pour the dressing over the quinoa salad and toss gently to coat.

6. Refrigerate the Greek•Style Quinoa Salad for at least 30 minutes to allow the flavors to blend.

7. Serve chilled or at room temperature.

This salad is high in fiber, protein, and healthy fats, making it a great option for people with diabetes. The combination of quinoa, vegetables, and feta cheese provides a satisfying and nutritious meal or side dish.

72. Greek•Style Stuffed Eggplant

Ingredient:

• 2 medium eggplants, halved lengthwise
• 1 tablespoon olive oil
• 1 onion, diced
• 2 cloves garlic, minced
• 1 cup diced tomatoes
• 1/2 cup cooked quinoa
• 1/4 cup crumbled feta cheese
• 2 tablespoons chopped fresh parsley
• 1 teaspoon dried oregano
• 1/4 teaspoon salt
• 1/4 teaspoon black pepper

Instructions:

1. Preheat your oven to 375°F (190°C).

2. Scoop out the flesh from the eggplant halves, leaving a 1/4•inch border. Chop the scooped•out eggplant flesh.

3. In a skillet, heat the olive oil over medium heat. Add the diced onion and chopped eggplant flesh, and sauté for 5•7 minutes, until the onion is translucent.

4. Add the minced garlic and cook for an additional 1•2 minutes, until fragrant.

5. Stir in the diced tomatoes, cooked quinoa, crumbled feta cheese, chopped parsley, dried oregano, salt, and black pepper. Mix well.

6. Spoon the quinoa mixture evenly into the hollowed•out eggplant halves.

7. Place the stuffed eggplant halves in a baking dish and bake for 25•30 minutes, or until the eggplant is tender and the filling is heated through.

8. Serve the Greek•Style Stuffed Eggplant warm.

This dish is a great way to incorporate more vegetables into your diet. The quinoa and feta cheese provide protein and healthy fats, making it a suitable option for people with diabetes.

73. Greek•Style Chicken Thighs

Ingredient:

• 8 bone•in, skin•on chicken thighs
• 2 tablespoons olive oil
• 2 tablespoons lemon juice
• 2 cloves garlic, minced
• 1 teaspoon dried oregano
• 1/2 teaspoon salt
• 1/4 teaspoon black pepper
• 1/4 cup crumbled feta cheese
• 2 tablespoons chopped fresh parsley

Instructions:

1. Preheat your oven to 400°F (200°C).

2. In a large bowl, combine the olive oil, lemon juice, minced garlic, dried oregano, salt, and black pepper. Add the chicken thighs and toss to coat them evenly with the marinade.

3. Arrange the marinated chicken thighs in a single layer on a baking sheet or in a large baking dish.

4. Bake the chicken in the preheated oven for 35•40 minutes, or until the chicken is cooked through and the skin is crispy.

5. Remove the chicken from the oven and sprinkle the crumbled feta cheese and chopped fresh parsley over the top.

6. Serve the Greek•Style Chicken Thighs immediately, while hot.

This dish is a great source of protein from the chicken, and the feta cheese provides a tangy, creamy element. The lemon, garlic, and oregano flavors complement the chicken beautifully, making this a delicious and healthy option for people with diabetes.

74. Greek•Style Green Beans

Ingredient:

- 1 lb fresh green beans, trimmed
- 2 tablespoons olive oil
- 2 cloves garlic, minced
- 1/4 cup crumbled feta cheese
- 2 tablespoons lemon juice
- 1 teaspoon dried oregano
- 1/4 teaspoon salt
- 1/4 teaspoon black pepper

Instructions:

1. Bring a large pot of salted water to a boil. Add the trimmed green beans and cook for 5•7 minutes, or until tender•crisp. Drain the green beans and set aside.

2. In a large skillet, heat the olive oil over medium heat. Add the minced garlic and cook for 1•2 minutes, stirring frequently, until fragrant.

3. Add the cooked green beans to the skillet with the garlic and olive oil. Toss to coat the beans evenly.

4. Remove the skillet from the heat and stir in the crumbled feta cheese, lemon juice, dried oregano, salt, and black pepper. Toss gently to combine.

5. Serve the Greek•Style Green Beans warm or at room temperature.

This dish is a simple and flavorful way to enjoy green beans. The feta cheese, lemon, and oregano give the green beans a Mediterranean•inspired taste. It's a great side dish that's low in carbs and high in fiber, making it a suitable option for people with diabetes.

75. Greek•Style Stuffed Squash

Ingredient:

- 4 small zucchini or yellow squash, halved lengthwise
- 1 tablespoon olive oil
- 1 onion, diced
- 2 cloves garlic, minced
- 1 cup cooked quinoa
- 1/2 cup crumbled feta cheese
- 1/4 cup chopped fresh parsley
- 1 tablespoon lemon juice
- 1 teaspoon dried oregano
- 1/4 teaspoon salt
- 1/4 teaspoon black pepper

Instructions:

1. Preheat your oven to 375°F (190°C).

2. Scoop out the seeds and flesh from the center of each squash half, leaving a 1/4•inch border. Chop the scooped•out flesh.

3. In a skillet, heat the olive oil over medium heat. Add the diced onion and chopped squash flesh, and sauté for 5•7 minutes, until the onion is translucent.

4. Add the minced garlic and cook for an additional 1•2 minutes, until fragrant.

5. Remove the skillet from the heat and stir in the cooked quinoa, crumbled feta cheese, chopped parsley, lemon juice, dried oregano, salt, and black pepper.

6. Spoon the quinoa mixture evenly into the hollowed•out squash halves.

7. Place the stuffed squash halves in a baking dish and bake for 20•25 minutes, or until the squash is tender and the filling is heated through.

8. Serve the Greek•Style Stuffed Squash warm.

This dish is a great way to incorporate more vegetables into your diet. The quinoa and feta cheese provide protein and healthy fats, making it a suitable option for people with diabetes.

76. Greek•Style Pork Chops

Ingredient:

• 4 (6 oz) boneless pork chops
• 2 tablespoons olive oil
• 2 tablespoons lemon juice
• 2 cloves garlic, minced
• 1 teaspoon dried oregano
• 1/2 teaspoon salt
• 1/4 teaspoon black pepper
• 1/4 cup crumbled feta cheese
• 2 tablespoons chopped fresh parsley

Instructions:

1. In a shallow dish or resealable plastic bag, combine the olive oil, lemon juice, minced garlic, dried oregano, salt, and black pepper. Add the pork chops and turn to coat them evenly with the marinade.

2. Cover the dish or seal the bag and refrigerate the pork chops for at least 30 minutes, or up to 4 hours, to allow the flavors to infuse.

3. Preheat your grill or grill pan to medium•high heat.

4. Remove the pork chops from the marinade and discard any remaining marinade.

5. Grill the pork chops for 4•6 minutes per side, or until they reach an internal temperature of 145°F (63°C).

6. Transfer the grilled pork chops to a serving plate and sprinkle the crumbled feta cheese and chopped fresh parsley over the top.

7. Serve the Greek•Style Pork Chops immediately, while hot.

This dish is a great source of protein from the pork, and the feta cheese provides a tangy, creamy element. The lemon, garlic, and oregano flavors complement the pork beautifully, making this a delicious and healthy option for people with diabetes.

77. Greek•Style Baked Halibut

Ingredient:

• 4 (6 oz) halibut fillets
• 2 tablespoons olive oil
• 2 tablespoons lemon juice
• 2 cloves garlic, minced
• 1 teaspoon dried oregano
• 1/2 teaspoon salt
• 1/4 teaspoon black pepper
• 1/4 cup crumbled feta cheese
• 2 tablespoons chopped fresh parsley

Instructions:

1. Preheat your oven to 400°F (200°C).

2. In a shallow baking dish or rimmed baking sheet, arrange the halibut fillets in a single layer.

3. In a small bowl, whisk together the olive oil, lemon juice, minced garlic, dried oregano, salt, and black pepper.

4. Drizzle the olive oil and lemon juice mixture over the halibut fillets, making sure to coat them evenly.

5. Bake the halibut in the preheated oven for 12•15 minutes, or until the fish flakes easily with a fork and is opaque throughout.

6. Remove the baked halibut from the oven and sprinkle the crumbled feta cheese and chopped fresh parsley over the top.

7. Serve the Greek•Style Baked Halibut immediately, while hot.

This dish is a great source of lean protein from the halibut, and the feta cheese provides a tangy, creamy element. The lemon, garlic, and oregano flavors complement the fish beautifully, making this a delicious and healthy option for people with diabetes.

78. Greek•Style Turkey Burgers

Ingredient:

• 1 lb ground turkey
• 1/4 cup crumbled feta cheese
• 2 tablespoons chopped fresh parsley
• 1 tablespoon lemon juice
• 1 teaspoon dried oregano
• 1/2 teaspoon salt
• 1/4 teaspoon black pepper
• 4 whole wheat burger buns
• Lettuce, tomato, and onion slices for serving (optional)

Instructions:

1. In a large bowl, combine the ground turkey, crumbled feta cheese, chopped parsley, lemon juice, dried oregano, salt, and black pepper. Mix well until the ingredients are evenly distributed.

2. Divide the turkey mixture into 4 equal portions and shape them into patties, each about 4 inches wide and 1/2 inch thick.

3. Preheat your grill or grill pan to medium•high heat.

4. Grill the turkey burgers for 4•6 minutes per side, or until they are cooked through and reach an internal temperature of 165°F (74°C).

5. Toast the whole wheat burger buns on the grill or in a toaster.

6. Place the grilled turkey burgers on the toasted buns. Top with lettuce, tomato, and onion slices, if desired.

7. Serve the Greek•Style Turkey Burgers immediately.

These burgers are a healthier alternative to traditional beef burgers, as they are made with lean ground turkey and packed with Mediterranean flavors from the feta cheese, parsley, and oregano. They are a great option for people with diabetes, as they are low in carbs and high in protein.

79. Greek•Style Shrimp Skewers

Ingredient:

• 1 lb large shrimp, peeled and deveined
• 2 tablespoons olive oil
• 2 tablespoons lemon juice
• 2 cloves garlic, minced
• 1 teaspoon dried oregano
• 1/4 teaspoon salt
• 1/4 teaspoon black pepper
• 1/4 cup crumbled feta cheese
• 2 tablespoons chopped fresh parsley

Instructions:

1. If using wooden skewers, soak them in water for 30 minutes to prevent them from burning.

2. In a large bowl, combine the shrimp, olive oil, lemon juice, minced garlic, dried oregano, salt, and black pepper. Toss to coat the shrimp evenly.

3. Thread the marinated shrimp onto the soaked skewers, leaving a small space between each shrimp.

4. Preheat your grill or grill pan to medium•high heat.

5. Grill the shrimp skewers for 2•3 minutes per side, or until the shrimp are opaque and cooked through.

6. Transfer the grilled shrimp skewers to a serving platter and sprinkle the crumbled feta cheese and chopped fresh parsley over the top.

7. Serve the Greek•Style Shrimp Skewers immediately, while hot.

This dish is a great source of lean protein from the shrimp, and the feta cheese provides a tangy, creamy element. The lemon, garlic, and oregano flavors complement the shrimp beautifully, making this a delicious and healthy option for people with diabetes.

80. Greek•Style Stuffed Cabbage

Ingredient:

• 1 medium head green cabbage
• 1 lb ground turkey
• 1/2 cup cooked quinoa
• 1/4 cup crumbled feta cheese
• 2 tablespoons chopped fresh parsley
• 1 teaspoon dried oregano
• 1/2 teaspoon salt
• 1/4 teaspoon black pepper
• 1 (15 oz) can diced tomatoes
• 1/4 cup water or low•sodium broth

Instructions:

1. Bring a large pot of water to a boil. Add the whole head of cabbage and cook for 5•7 minutes, until the outer leaves are softened. Remove the cabbage from the water and let it cool slightly.

2. Carefully peel off the softened cabbage leaves, one at a time, and set them aside. Chop any remaining cabbage that is too small to stuff.

3. In a large bowl, combine the ground turkey, cooked quinoa, crumbled feta cheese, chopped parsley, dried oregano, salt, and black pepper. Mix well.

4. Place a heaping spoonful of the turkey mixture onto the center of each cabbage leaf. Fold the sides of the leaf over the filling and then roll up the leaf to completely enclose the filling.

5. Arrange the stuffed cabbage rolls in a baking dish. Pour the diced tomatoes and water or broth over the top.

6. Cover the baking dish and bake at 375°F (190°C) for 45•55 minutes, or until the cabbage is tender and the filling is cooked through. Serve the Greek•Style Stuffed Cabbage warm.

This dish is a great way to incorporate more vegetables and lean protein into your diet. The feta cheese and Mediterranean herbs add a delicious flavor, making it a suitable option for people with diabetes.

81. Greek•Style Roasted Cauliflower

Ingredient:

- 1 head of cauliflower, cut into florets
- 2 tablespoons olive oil
- 2 cloves garlic, minced
- 1 teaspoon dried oregano
- 1/2 teaspoon salt
- 1/4 teaspoon black pepper
- 1/4 cup crumbled feta cheese
- 2 tablespoons chopped fresh parsley

Instructions:

1. Preheat your oven to 400°F (200°C).

2. In a large bowl, toss the cauliflower florets with the olive oil, minced garlic, dried oregano, salt, and black pepper until the cauliflower is evenly coated.

3. Spread the seasoned cauliflower in a single layer on a baking sheet.

4. Roast the cauliflower in the preheated oven for 20•25 minutes, or until it is tender and lightly browned, stirring halfway through.

5. Remove the roasted cauliflower from the oven and sprinkle the crumbled feta cheese and chopped fresh parsley over the top.

6. Serve the Greek•Style Roasted Cauliflower warm.

This dish is a simple and flavorful way to enjoy cauliflower. The feta cheese provides a tangy, creamy element, while the oregano and garlic add a Mediterranean flavor. It's a great low•carb side dish that's suitable for people with diabetes.

82. Greek•Style Broccoli Rabe

Ingredient:

• 1 lb broccoli rabe, trimmed and chopped
• 2 tablespoons olive oil
• 2 cloves garlic, minced
• 1 tablespoon lemon juice
• 1 teaspoon dried oregano
• 1/4 teaspoon salt
• 1/4 teaspoon black pepper
• 2 tablespoons crumbled feta cheese
• 1 tablespoon chopped fresh parsley

Instructions:

1. Bring a large pot of salted water to a boil. Add the chopped broccoli rabe and blanch for 2•3 minutes, until tender•crisp. Drain the broccoli rabe and set aside.

2. In a large skillet, heat the olive oil over medium heat. Add the minced garlic and cook for 1•2 minutes, until fragrant.

3. Add the blanched broccoli rabe to the skillet with the garlic and olive oil. Drizzle the lemon juice over the top and sprinkle with the dried oregano, salt, and black pepper.

4. Sauté the broccoli rabe for 3•5 minutes, stirring frequently, until it is tender and the flavors have melded.

5. Remove the skillet from the heat and sprinkle the crumbled feta cheese and chopped fresh parsley over the broccoli rabe.

6. Serve the Greek•Style Broccoli Rabe warm.

This dish is a great way to incorporate more leafy greens into your diet. The feta cheese, lemon, and oregano provide a Mediterranean•inspired flavor that complements the broccoli rabe perfectly. It's a suitable option for people with diabetes.

83. Greek•Style Chicken Wings

Ingredient:

• 2 lbs chicken wings, drumettes and flats separated
• 2 tablespoons olive oil
• 2 tablespoons lemon juice
• 2 cloves garlic, minced
• 1 teaspoon dried oregano
• 1/2 teaspoon salt
• 1/4 teaspoon black pepper
• 1/4 cup crumbled feta cheese
• 2 tablespoons chopped fresh parsley

Instructions:

1. Preheat your oven to 400°F (200°C).

2. In a large bowl, combine the chicken wings, olive oil, lemon juice, minced garlic, dried oregano, salt, and black pepper. Toss to coat the wings evenly.

3. Arrange the seasoned chicken wings in a single layer on a baking sheet or in a large baking dish.

4. Bake the chicken wings in the preheated oven for 35•40 minutes, flipping them halfway through, until they are crispy and cooked through.

5. Remove the baked chicken wings from the oven and sprinkle the crumbled feta cheese and chopped fresh parsley over the top.

6. Serve the Greek•Style Chicken Wings immediately, while hot.

These chicken wings are a delicious and healthy option for people with diabetes. The lemon, garlic, and oregano flavors provide a Mediterranean twist, while the feta cheese adds a tangy, creamy element. This dish is a great source of protein and can be enjoyed as an appetizer or a main course.

84. Greek•Style Stuffed Chicken Breast

Ingredient:

• 4 (6 oz) boneless, skinless chicken breasts
• 1/2 cup crumbled feta cheese
• 2 tablespoons chopped fresh spinach
• 1 tablespoon chopped fresh parsley
• 1 teaspoon dried oregano
• 1/4 teaspoon salt
• 1/4 teaspoon black pepper
• 1 tablespoon olive oil

Instructions:

1. Preheat your oven to 400°F (200°C).

2. Use a sharp knife to cut a pocket into the side of each chicken breast, being careful not to cut all the way through.

3. In a small bowl, mix together the crumbled feta cheese, chopped spinach, chopped parsley, dried oregano, salt, and black pepper.

4. Stuff the feta cheese mixture evenly into the pockets of the chicken breasts.

5. Heat the olive oil in a large oven•safe skillet over medium•high heat.

6. Add the stuffed chicken breasts to the skillet and sear for 2•3 minutes per side, or until the outside is lightly browned.

7. Transfer the skillet to the preheated oven and bake the chicken for 20•25 minutes, or until the chicken is cooked through and the internal temperature reaches 165°F (74°C).

8. Remove the Greek•Style Stuffed Chicken Breast from the oven and let it rest for a few minutes before serving.

This dish is a great way to add more protein and healthy fats to your diet. The feta cheese, spinach, and herbs provide a delicious Mediterranean flavor that is suitable for people with diabetes.

85. Greek•Style Garlic Bread

Ingredient:

• 1 whole wheat baguette, sliced into 1•inch thick pieces
• 2 tablespoons olive oil
• 2 cloves garlic, minced
• 1 teaspoon dried oregano
• 1/4 teaspoon salt
• 1/4 teaspoon black pepper
• 2 tablespoons crumbled feta cheese
• 1 tablespoon chopped fresh parsley

Instructions:

1. Preheat your oven to 400°F (200°C).

2. In a small bowl, combine the olive oil, minced garlic, dried oregano, salt, and black pepper. Stir to mix well.

3. Arrange the sliced baguette pieces on a baking sheet.

4. Brush the garlic•herb oil mixture evenly over the top of the baguette slices.

5. Bake the garlic bread in the preheated oven for 8•10 minutes, or until the bread is lightly toasted and the edges are crispy.

6. Remove the garlic bread from the oven and sprinkle the crumbled feta cheese and chopped fresh parsley over the top.

7. Serve the Greek•Style Garlic Bread warm.

This garlic bread is a healthier alternative to traditional versions, as it uses whole wheat bread and incorporates Mediterranean flavors from the feta cheese, oregano, and parsley. It's a great side dish that's suitable for people with diabetes, as it's low in carbs and high in flavor.

86. Greek•Style Tuna Casserole

Ingredient:

• 2 (5 oz) cans tuna, drained and flaked
• 1 cup cooked quinoa
• 1 cup diced tomatoes
• 1/2 cup crumbled feta cheese
• 1/4 cup sliced black olives
• 2 tablespoons chopped fresh parsley
• 1 tablespoon lemon juice
• 1 teaspoon dried oregano
• 1/4 teaspoon salt
• 1/4 teaspoon black pepper
• 1/4 cup whole wheat breadcrumbs

Instructions:

1. Preheat your oven to 375°F (190°C).

2. In a large bowl, combine the flaked tuna, cooked quinoa, diced tomatoes, crumbled feta cheese, sliced black olives, chopped parsley, lemon juice, dried oregano, salt, and black pepper. Mix well.

3. Transfer the tuna and quinoa mixture to a 9x13 inch baking dish.

4. Sprinkle the whole wheat breadcrumbs evenly over the top of the casserole.

5. Bake the Greek•Style Tuna Casserole in the preheated oven for 20•25 minutes, or until the breadcrumbs are golden brown and the casserole is heated through.

6. Remove the casserole from the oven and let it cool for a few minutes before serving.

7. Serve the Greek•Style Tuna Casserole warm.

This casserole is a great way to incorporate more protein, fiber, and healthy fats into your diet. The tuna, quinoa, and feta cheese provide a nutritious and satisfying meal that is suitable for people with diabetes.

87. Greek•Style Baked Scallops

Ingredient:

- 1 lb sea scallops, patted dry
- 2 tablespoons olive oil
- 2 tablespoons lemon juice
- 2 cloves garlic, minced
- 1 teaspoon dried oregano
- 1/4 teaspoon salt
- 1/4 teaspoon black pepper
- 1/4 cup crumbled feta cheese
- 2 tablespoons chopped fresh parsley

Instructions:

1. Preheat your oven to 400°F (200°C).

2. In a large bowl, combine the scallops, olive oil, lemon juice, minced garlic, dried oregano, salt, and black pepper. Toss to coat the scallops evenly.

3. Arrange the seasoned scallops in a single layer in a baking dish or on a rimmed baking sheet.

4. Bake the scallops in the preheated oven for 10•12 minutes, or until they are opaque and cooked through.

5. Remove the baked scallops from the oven and sprinkle the crumbled feta cheese and chopped fresh parsley over the top.

6. Serve the Greek•Style Baked Scallops immediately, while hot.

This dish is a great source of lean protein from the scallops, and the feta cheese provides a tangy, creamy element. The lemon, garlic, and oregano flavors complement the scallops beautifully, making this a delicious and healthy option for people with diabetes.

88. Greek•Style Roasted Asparagus

Ingredient:

- 1 lb asparagus, trimmed
- 2 tablespoons olive oil
- 2 cloves garlic, minced
- 1 teaspoon dried oregano
- 1/4 teaspoon salt
- 1/4 teaspoon black pepper
- 2 tablespoons crumbled feta cheese
- 1 tablespoon chopped fresh parsley

Instructions:

1. Preheat your oven to 400°F (200°C).

2. In a large bowl, toss the trimmed asparagus with the olive oil, minced garlic, dried oregano, salt, and black pepper until the asparagus is evenly coated.

3. Spread the seasoned asparagus in a single layer on a baking sheet.

4. Roast the asparagus in the preheated oven for 12•15 minutes, or until it is tender and lightly browned, stirring halfway through.

5. Remove the roasted asparagus from the oven and sprinkle the crumbled feta cheese and chopped fresh parsley over the top.

6. Serve the Greek•Style Roasted Asparagus warm.

This dish is a simple and flavorful way to enjoy asparagus. The feta cheese provides a tangy, creamy element, while the oregano and garlic add a Mediterranean flavor. It's a great low•carb side dish that's suitable for people with diabetes.

89. Greek•Style Baked Pork Chops

Ingredient:

• 4 (6 oz) boneless pork chops
• 2 tablespoons olive oil
• 2 tablespoons lemon juice
• 2 cloves garlic, minced
• 1 teaspoon dried oregano
• 1/2 teaspoon salt
• 1/4 teaspoon black pepper
• 1/4 cup crumbled feta cheese
• 2 tablespoons chopped fresh parsley

Instructions:

1. Preheat your oven to 400°F (200°C).

2. In a shallow baking dish or rimmed baking sheet, arrange the pork chops in a single layer.

3. In a small bowl, whisk together the olive oil, lemon juice, minced garlic, dried oregano, salt, and black pepper.

4. Drizzle the olive oil and lemon juice mixture over the pork chops, making sure to coat them evenly.

5. Bake the pork chops in the preheated oven for 20•25 minutes, or until they reach an internal temperature of 145°F (63°C).

6. Remove the baked pork chops from the oven and sprinkle the crumbled feta cheese and chopped fresh parsley over the top.

7. Serve the Greek•Style Baked Pork Chops immediately, while hot.

This dish is a great source of lean protein from the pork, and the feta cheese provides a tangy, creamy element. The lemon, garlic, and oregano flavors complement the pork beautifully, making this a delicious and healthy option for people with diabetes.

90. Greek•Style Brussels Sprouts Salad

Ingredient:

- 1 lb Brussels sprouts, trimmed and shredded
- 1/4 cup crumbled feta cheese
- 1/4 cup sliced kalamata olives
- 2 tablespoons chopped fresh parsley
- 2 tablespoons lemon juice
- 1 tablespoon olive oil
- 1 teaspoon dried oregano
- 1/4 teaspoon salt
- 1/4 teaspoon black pepper

Instructions:

1. In a large bowl, combine the shredded Brussels sprouts, crumbled feta cheese, sliced kalamata olives, and chopped fresh parsley.

2. In a small bowl, whisk together the lemon juice, olive oil, dried oregano, salt, and black pepper.

3. Pour the dressing over the Brussels sprouts mixture and toss gently to coat.

4. Cover the salad and refrigerate for at least 30 minutes to allow the flavors to blend.

5. Serve the Greek•Style Brussels Sprouts Salad chilled or at room temperature.

This salad is a great way to incorporate more cruciferous vegetables into your diet. The Brussels sprouts provide fiber and important nutrients, while the feta cheese, olives, and Mediterranean•inspired dressing add flavor and healthy fats. It's a suitable option for people with diabetes.

91. Greek•Style Baked Zucchini

Ingredient:

• 3 medium zucchini, sliced into 1/2•inch rounds
• 2 tablespoons olive oil
• 2 cloves garlic, minced
• 1 teaspoon dried oregano
• 1/2 teaspoon salt
• 1/4 teaspoon black pepper
• 1/2 cup crumbled feta cheese
• 2 tablespoons chopped fresh parsley

Instructions:

1. Preheat your oven to 400°F (200°C).

2. In a large bowl, toss the zucchini slices with the olive oil, minced garlic, dried oregano, salt, and black pepper until the zucchini is evenly coated.

3. Arrange the seasoned zucchini slices in a single layer on a baking sheet or in a large baking dish.

4. Bake the zucchini in the preheated oven for 15•20 minutes, or until the zucchini is tender and lightly browned.

5. Remove the baked zucchini from the oven and sprinkle the crumbled feta cheese and chopped fresh parsley over the top.

6. Serve the Greek•Style Baked Zucchini warm.

This dish is a great way to incorporate more vegetables into your diet. The feta cheese provides a tangy, creamy element, while the oregano and garlic add a Mediterranean flavor. It's a simple and delicious side dish that's suitable for people with diabetes.

92. Greek•Style Green Salad with Chicken

Ingredient:

• 6 cups mixed greens (such as spinach, arugula, and romaine)
• 1 cup cooked and shredded chicken breast
• 1/2 cup cherry tomatoes, halved
• 1/4 cup crumbled feta cheese
• 2 tablespoons sliced kalamata olives
• 2 tablespoons chopped fresh parsley
• 2 tablespoons lemon juice
• 1 tablespoon olive oil
• 1 teaspoon dried oregano
• 1/4 teaspoon salt
• 1/4 teaspoon black pepper

Instructions:

1. In a large salad bowl, combine the mixed greens, shredded chicken, cherry tomatoes, crumbled feta cheese, sliced kalamata olives, and chopped fresh parsley.

2. In a small bowl, whisk together the lemon juice, olive oil, dried oregano, salt, and black pepper to make the dressing.

3. Pour the dressing over the salad and toss gently to coat the ingredients evenly.

4. Serve the Greek•Style Green Salad with Chicken immediately.

This salad is a great way to incorporate lean protein, healthy fats, and a variety of nutrient•dense vegetables into your diet. The Mediterranean•inspired flavors from the feta cheese, olives, and oregano make it a delicious and satisfying option for people with diabetes.

93. Greek•Style Stuffed Bell Peppers

Ingredient:

• 4 medium bell peppers, halved and seeded
• 1 lb ground turkey
• 1 cup cooked quinoa
• 1/2 cup crumbled feta cheese
• 1/4 cup chopped fresh parsley
• 2 cloves garlic, minced
• 1 teaspoon dried oregano
• 1/4 teaspoon salt
• 1/4 teaspoon black pepper
• 1 (14.5 oz) can diced tomatoes

Instructions:

1. Preheat your oven to 375°F (190°C).

2. Arrange the bell pepper halves in a baking dish or on a rimmed baking sheet.

3. In a large bowl, combine the ground turkey, cooked quinoa, crumbled feta cheese, chopped parsley, minced garlic, dried oregano, salt, and black pepper. Mix well.

4. Spoon the turkey and quinoa mixture evenly into the bell pepper halves.

5. Pour the diced tomatoes around the stuffed peppers in the baking dish.

6. Cover the baking dish with foil and bake for 30•35 minutes, or until the peppers are tender and the filling is cooked through.

7. Remove the foil and bake for an additional 5•10 minutes, or until the tops of the stuffed peppers are lightly browned.

8. Serve the Greek•Style Stuffed Bell Peppers warm.

This dish is a great way to incorporate more vegetables, protein, and healthy grains into your diet. The feta cheese and Mediterranean•inspired flavors make it a suitable option for people with diabetes.

94. Greek•Style Grilled Lamb

Ingredient:

• 1 lb lamb loin chops or leg of lamb, cut into 1•inch cubes
• 2 tablespoons olive oil
• 2 tablespoons lemon juice
• 2 cloves garlic, minced
• 1 teaspoon dried oregano
• 1/2 teaspoon salt
• 1/4 teaspoon black pepper
• 2 tablespoons crumbled feta cheese
• 2 tablespoons chopped fresh parsley

Instructions:

1. In a large bowl, combine the lamb cubes, olive oil, lemon juice, minced garlic, dried oregano, salt, and black pepper. Toss to coat the lamb evenly.

2. Thread the marinated lamb cubes onto metal or wooden skewers.

3. Preheat your grill or grill pan to medium•high heat.

4. Grill the lamb skewers for 8•10 minutes, turning occasionally, until the lamb is cooked to your desired doneness.

5. Transfer the grilled Greek•Style Lamb Skewers to a serving platter.

6. Sprinkle the crumbled feta cheese and chopped fresh parsley over the top of the lamb.

7. Serve the Greek•Style Grilled Lamb immediately, while hot.

This dish is a great source of lean protein from the lamb, and the feta cheese provides a tangy, creamy element. The lemon, garlic, and oregano flavors complement the lamb beautifully, making this a delicious and healthy option for people with diabetes.

95. Greek•Style Spaghetti Squash Salad

Ingredient:

- 1 medium spaghetti squash, halved and seeded
- 2 tablespoons olive oil
- 1 tablespoon lemon juice
- 1 teaspoon dried oregano
- 1/4 teaspoon salt
- 1/4 teaspoon black pepper
- 1/2 cup cherry tomatoes, halved
- 1/4 cup crumbled feta cheese
- 2 tablespoons sliced kalamata olives
- 2 tablespoons chopped fresh parsley

Instructions:

1. Preheat your oven to 400°F (200°C).

2. Place the spaghetti squash halves cut•side down on a baking sheet. Bake for 30•40 minutes, or until the squash is tender and easily shreds with a fork.

3. Remove the spaghetti squash from the oven and let it cool slightly. Use a fork to shred the flesh into spaghetti•like strands and transfer them to a large bowl.

4. In a small bowl, whisk together the olive oil, lemon juice, dried oregano, salt, and black pepper.

5. Pour the dressing over the shredded spaghetti squash and toss to coat.

6. Add the cherry tomatoes, crumbled feta cheese, sliced kalamata olives, and chopped fresh parsley to the bowl. Gently toss to combine.

7. Serve the Greek•Style Spaghetti Squash Salad chilled or at room temperature.

This salad is a great low•carb option that's packed with flavor from the Mediterranean•inspired ingredients. The spaghetti squash provides fiber, while the feta cheese and olives add healthy fats, making it a suitable choice for people with diabetes.

96. Greek•Style Stuffed Chicken Thighs

Ingredient:

• 8 boneless, skinless chicken thighs
• 1/2 cup crumbled feta cheese
• 1/4 cup chopped fresh spinach
• 2 tbsp chopped fresh parsley
• 1 clove garlic, minced
• 1 tsp dried oregano
• 1/4 tsp salt
• 1/4 tsp black pepper
• 1 tbsp olive oil

Instructions:

1. Preheat oven to 400°F. Lightly grease a baking dish.

2. In a small bowl, mix together the feta cheese, spinach, parsley, garlic, oregano, salt, and pepper.

3. Carefully slice each chicken thigh horizontally to create a pocket, being careful not to cut all the way through.

4. Stuff each chicken thigh with about 2 tbsp of the feta•spinach mixture.

5. Place the stuffed chicken thighs in the prepared baking dish and drizzle with the olive oil.

6. Bake for 30•35 minutes, or until the chicken is cooked through and reaches an internal temperature of 165°F.

7. Serve immediately.

These Greek•style stuffed chicken thighs are a delicious and healthy option for people with diabetes. The feta cheese and spinach filling adds flavor and nutrients, while the chicken thighs provide a good source of lean protein. This dish is low in carbs and high in healthy fats and protein, making it a great choice for a diabetes•friendly meal.

97. Greek•Style Baked Trout

Ingredient:

• 4 trout fillets (about 1 lb total)
• 2 tbsp olive oil
• 2 tbsp lemon juice
• 2 cloves garlic, minced
• 1 tsp dried oregano
• 1/4 tsp salt
• 1/4 tsp black pepper
• 1/2 cup crumbled feta cheese
• 2 tbsp chopped fresh parsley

Instructions:

1. Preheat oven to 400°F. Lightly grease a baking dish.

2. In a small bowl, whisk together the olive oil, lemon juice, garlic, oregano, salt, and pepper.

3. Place the trout fillets in the prepared baking dish. Pour the lemon•garlic mixture over the top, making sure to coat the fish evenly.

4. Sprinkle the crumbled feta cheese over the top of the fillets.

5. Bake for 15•20 minutes, or until the fish flakes easily with a fork and reaches an internal temperature of 145°F.

6. Remove from oven and sprinkle with chopped fresh parsley.

7. Serve immediately.

This Greek•style baked trout is a delicious and healthy option for people with diabetes. Trout is a lean, high•protein fish that is also a good source of heart•healthy omega•3 fatty acids. The feta cheese and herbs add flavor without adding too many carbs.

98. Greek•Style Roasted Bell Peppers

Ingredient:

• 4 large bell peppers (mix of red, yellow, and orange)
• 2 tbsp olive oil
• 2 cloves garlic, minced
• 1 tsp dried oregano
• 1/4 tsp salt
• 1/4 tsp black pepper
• 1/4 cup crumbled feta cheese
• 2 tbsp chopped fresh parsley

Instructions:

1. Preheat oven to 400°F. Line a baking sheet with parchment paper.

2. Cut the bell peppers in half lengthwise and remove the seeds and membranes. Place the pepper halves cut•side up on the prepared baking sheet.

3. In a small bowl, whisk together the olive oil, garlic, oregano, salt, and pepper.

4. Brush the cut side of the peppers with the garlic•oil mixture, making sure to coat them evenly.

5. Roast the peppers for 25•30 minutes, or until they are tender and slightly charred on the edges.

6. Remove the peppers from the oven and sprinkle the crumbled feta cheese over the top.

7. Return the peppers to the oven and bake for an additional 5 minutes, or until the feta is melted.

8. Garnish with chopped fresh parsley before serving.

These Greek•style roasted bell peppers are a delicious and healthy side dish that is suitable for people with diabetes. The peppers are roasted to bring out their natural sweetness, and the feta cheese and herbs add a flavorful Mediterranean twist. This dish is low in carbs and high in fiber, vitamins, and antioxidants.

99. Greek•Style Stuffed Cucumbers

Ingredient:

• 4 medium cucumbers
• 1 cup crumbled feta cheese
• 1/4 cup chopped fresh dill
• 2 tbsp chopped fresh parsley
• 1 clove garlic, minced
• 1 tbsp lemon juice
• 1/4 tsp salt
• 1/4 tsp black pepper

Instructions:

1. Cut the cucumbers in half lengthwise and use a spoon to scoop out the seeds, creating a boat•like shape.

2. In a medium bowl, mix together the feta cheese, dill, parsley, garlic, lemon juice, salt, and pepper until well combined.

3. Spoon the feta mixture evenly into the hollowed•out cucumber halves.

4. Arrange the stuffed cucumber halves on a serving platter.

5. Refrigerate for at least 30 minutes to allow the flavors to meld. Serve chilled.

Nutritional Information (per serving):
Calories: 80
Total Fat: 5g
Saturated Fat: 3g
Cholesterol: 15mg
Sodium: 260mg
Total Carbs: 5g
Fiber: 1g
Sugars: 2g
Protein: 5g

These Greek•style stuffed cucumbers are a refreshing and healthy appetizer or side dish that is perfect for people with diabetes. The creamy feta cheese filling is balanced by the crisp, hydrating cucumber. This dish is low in carbs, high in fiber, and provides a good source of protein. It's a great option for a diabetes•friendly snack or light meal.

100. Greek•Style Turkey Meatloaf

Ingredient:

- 1 lb ground turkey
- 1 cup whole wheat breadcrumbs
- 1/2 cup crumbled feta cheese
- 1/4 cup chopped fresh parsley
- 2 cloves garlic, minced
- 1 egg, lightly beaten
- 1 tsp dried oregano
- 1/4 tsp salt
- 1/4 tsp black pepper

Instructions:

1. Preheat oven to 375°F. Lightly grease a 9x5 inch loaf pan.

2. In a large bowl, combine the ground turkey, breadcrumbs, feta cheese, parsley, garlic, egg, oregano, salt, and pepper. Mix well until all ingredients are evenly distributed.

3. Transfer the mixture to the prepared loaf pan and shape into a loaf.

4. Bake for 50•60 minutes, or until the internal temperature reaches 165°F.

5. Let the meatloaf rest for 5•10 minutes before slicing and serving.

Nutritional Information (per serving):
Calories: 200
Total Fat: 9g
Saturated Fat: 3g
Cholesterol: 95mg
Sodium: 380mg
Total Carbs: 12g
Fiber: 2g
Sugars: 1g
Protein: 22g

This turkey meatloaf is a healthier alternative to traditional beef meatloaf. The feta cheese and herbs add a delicious Greek•inspired flavor. It's a great option for people with diabetes as it's high in protein, moderate in carbs, and low in saturated fat.

101. Greek•Style Baked Tilapia

Ingredient:

• 4 tilapia fillets (about 1 lb total)
• 2 tbsp olive oil
• 2 tbsp lemon juice
• 2 cloves garlic, minced
• 1 tsp dried oregano
• 1/4 tsp salt
• 1/4 tsp black pepper
• 1/2 cup crumbled feta cheese
• 2 tbsp chopped fresh parsley

Instructions:

1. Preheat oven to 400°F. Lightly grease a baking dish.

2. In a small bowl, whisk together the olive oil, lemon juice, garlic, oregano, salt, and pepper.

3. Place the tilapia fillets in the prepared baking dish. Pour the lemon•garlic mixture over the top, making sure to coat the fish evenly.

4. Sprinkle the crumbled feta cheese over the top of the fillets.

5. Bake for 15•20 minutes, or until the fish flakes easily with a fork and reaches an internal temperature of 145°F.

6. Remove from oven and sprinkle with chopped fresh parsley.

7. Serve immediately.

This Greek•style baked tilapia is a delicious and healthy option for people with diabetes. Tilapia is a lean, mild•flavored fish that is a good source of protein. The feta cheese and herbs add a Mediterranean twist without adding too many carbs. This dish is low in calories and carbs, making it a great choice for a diabetes•friendly meal.

102. Greek•Style Stuffed Mushrooms

Ingredient:

• 12 large mushrooms, stems removed and finely chopped
• 2 tbsp olive oil
• 1/4 cup finely chopped onion
• 2 cloves garlic, minced
• 1/4 cup crumbled feta cheese
• 2 tbsp chopped fresh parsley
• 1 tsp dried oregano
• 1/4 tsp salt
• 1/4 tsp black pepper

Instructions:

1. Preheat oven to 375°F. Lightly grease a baking sheet.

2. In a skillet, heat the olive oil over medium heat. Add the chopped mushroom stems, onion, and garlic. Sauté for 5•7 minutes, until the vegetables are softened.

3. Remove the skillet from heat and stir in the feta cheese, parsley, oregano, salt, and pepper. Mix well.

4. Stuff the mushroom caps with the feta•mushroom mixture, packing it in tightly.

5. Arrange the stuffed mushrooms on the prepared baking sheet.

6. Bake for 15•20 minutes, or until the mushrooms are tender and the filling is heated through. Serve warm.

Nutritional Information (per serving):
Calories: 50
Total Fat: 3g
Saturated Fat: 1g
Cholesterol: 5mg

These Greek•style stuffed mushrooms are a delicious and diabetes•friendly appetizer or snack. The feta cheese, herbs, and sautéed mushroom stems create a flavorful filling that complements the earthy mushroom caps. This recipe is low in carbs and calories, making it a great option for people with diabetes.

103. Greek•Style Chicken Drumsticks

Ingredient:

- 8 chicken drumsticks
- 2 tablespoons olive oil
- 2 tablespoons lemon juice
- 2 cloves garlic, minced
- 1 teaspoon dried oregano
- 1/2 teaspoon salt
- 1/4 teaspoon black pepper
- 1/4 cup crumbled feta cheese
- 2 tablespoons chopped fresh parsley

Instructions:

1. Preheat your oven to 400°F (200°C).

2. In a large bowl, combine the chicken drumsticks, olive oil, lemon juice, minced garlic, dried oregano, salt, and black pepper. Toss to coat the drumsticks evenly.

3. Arrange the seasoned chicken drumsticks in a single layer on a baking sheet or in a large baking dish.

4. Bake the chicken in the preheated oven for 35•40 minutes, or until the drumsticks are cooked through and the skin is crispy, turning them halfway through.

5. Remove the baked chicken drumsticks from the oven and sprinkle the crumbled feta cheese and chopped fresh parsley over the top.

6. Serve the Greek•Style Chicken Drumsticks immediately, while hot.

This dish is a great source of protein from the chicken, and the feta cheese provides a tangy, creamy element. The lemon, garlic, and oregano flavors complement the chicken beautifully, making this a delicious and healthy option for people with diabetes.

104. Greek•Style Stuffed Pork Tenderloin

Ingredient:

- 1 lb pork tenderloin
- 1/2 cup crumbled feta cheese
- 1/4 cup chopped fresh spinach
- 2 tbsp chopped fresh parsley
- 1 clove garlic, minced
- 1 tsp dried oregano
- 1/4 tsp salt
- 1/4 tsp black pepper
- 1 tbsp olive oil

Instructions:

1. Preheat oven to 400°F. Lightly grease a baking dish.

2. Slice the pork tenderloin lengthwise, being careful not to cut all the way through, to create a pocket.

3. In a small bowl, mix together the feta cheese, spinach, parsley, garlic, oregano, salt, and pepper.

4. Stuff the feta•spinach mixture into the pocket of the pork tenderloin.

5. Tie the tenderloin with kitchen string to help it hold its shape.

6. Place the stuffed pork tenderloin in the prepared baking dish and drizzle with the olive oil.

7. Bake for 30•35 minutes, or until the pork is cooked through and reaches an internal temperature of 145°F. Let the pork rest for 5•10 minutes before slicing and serving.

Nutritional Information (per serving):
Calories: 220
Total Fat: 10g

This Greek•style stuffed pork tenderloin is a delicious and diabetes•friendly main dish. Pork tenderloin is a lean protein that is high in nutrients. The feta cheese and spinach filling adds flavor and moisture to the pork, while the herbs provide a Mediterranean flair. This dish is low in carbs and high in protein, making it a great option for people with diabetes.

105. Greek·Style Baked Sweet Potatoes

Ingredient:

• 4 medium sweet potatoes, scrubbed clean
• 2 tbsp olive oil
• 2 tbsp lemon juice
• 2 cloves garlic, minced
• 1 tsp dried oregano
• 1/4 tsp salt
• 1/4 tsp black pepper
• 1/2 cup crumbled feta cheese
• 2 tbsp chopped fresh parsley

Instructions:

1. Preheat oven to 400°F. Pierce the sweet potatoes several times with a fork.

2. Bake the sweet potatoes for 45·60 minutes, or until they are tender when pierced with a fork.

3. In a small bowl, whisk together the olive oil, lemon juice, garlic, oregano, salt, and pepper.

4. Once the sweet potatoes are cooked, slice them open lengthwise. Drizzle the lemon·garlic mixture over the top.

5. Sprinkle the crumbled feta cheese and chopped fresh parsley over the sweet potatoes. Serve warm.

Nutritional Information (per serving):
Calories: 180
Total Fat: 7g
Saturated Fat: 3g
Cholesterol: 15mg

These Greek·style baked sweet potatoes are a delicious and diabetes·friendly side dish. Sweet potatoes are a nutrient·dense carbohydrate that is high in fiber and vitamins. The feta cheese and herbs add a Mediterranean flavor without adding too many additional carbs. This dish is a great option for people with diabetes who are looking for a flavorful and healthy way to enjoy sweet potatoes.

106. Greek•Style Stuffed Cod

Ingredient:

• 4 cod fillets (about 1 lb total)
• 1/2 cup crumbled feta cheese
• 1/4 cup chopped fresh spinach
• 2 tbsp chopped fresh parsley
• 1 clove garlic, minced
• 1 tsp dried oregano
• 1/4 tsp salt
• 1/4 tsp black pepper
• 1 tbsp olive oil

Instructions:

1. Preheat oven to 400°F. Lightly grease a baking dish.

2. Carefully slice each cod fillet horizontally to create a pocket, being careful not to cut all the way through.

3. In a small bowl, mix together the feta cheese, spinach, parsley, garlic, oregano, salt, and pepper.

4. Stuff the feta•spinach mixture into the pockets of the cod fillets.

5. Place the stuffed cod fillets in the prepared baking dish and drizzle with the olive oil.

6. Bake for 18•22 minutes, or until the cod is cooked through and flakes easily with a fork. Serve immediately.

Nutritional Information (per serving):
Calories: 200
Total Fat: 9g
Saturated Fat: 3g

This Greek•style stuffed cod is a delicious and diabetes•friendly main dish. Cod is a lean, flaky fish that is high in protein and low in carbs. The feta cheese and spinach filling adds flavor and moisture to the fish, while the herbs provide a Mediterranean flair. This dish is a great option for people with diabetes who are looking for a healthy and flavorful seafood meal.

107. Greek•Style Grilled Swordfish

Ingredient:

• 4 swordfish steaks (about 1 lb total)
• 2 tbsp olive oil
• 2 tbsp lemon juice
• 2 cloves garlic, minced
• 1 tsp dried oregano
• 1/4 tsp salt
• 1/4 tsp black pepper
• 1/4 cup crumbled feta cheese
• 2 tbsp chopped fresh parsley

Instructions:

1. Preheat grill or grill pan to medium•high heat.

2. In a shallow dish, whisk together the olive oil, lemon juice, garlic, oregano, salt, and pepper.

3. Add the swordfish steaks to the dish and turn to coat both sides with the marinade.

4. Grill the swordfish for 4•5 minutes per side, or until it flakes easily with a fork and reaches an internal temperature of 145°F.

5. Transfer the grilled swordfish to a serving platter.

6. Sprinkle the crumbled feta cheese and chopped fresh parsley over the top.

7. Serve immediately.

Nutritional Information (per serving):
Calories: 220
Total Fat: 10g
Saturated Fat: 3g

This Greek•style grilled swordfish is a delicious and diabetes•friendly main dish. Swordfish is a lean, high•protein fish that is also a good source of omega•3 fatty acids. The feta cheese and herbs add a Mediterranean flavor without adding too many carbs. This dish is low in carbs and high in protein, making it a great option for people with diabetes.

108. Greek•Style Baked Chicken Thighs

Ingredient:

• 8 bone•in, skin•on chicken thighs
• 2 tbsp olive oil
• 2 tbsp lemon juice
• 2 cloves garlic, minced
• 1 tsp dried oregano
• 1/2 tsp salt
• 1/4 tsp black pepper
• 1/2 cup crumbled feta cheese
• 2 tbsp chopped fresh parsley

Instructions:

1. Preheat oven to 400°F. Lightly grease a baking dish.

2. In a small bowl, whisk together the olive oil, lemon juice, garlic, oregano, salt, and pepper.

3. Place the chicken thighs in the prepared baking dish and pour the lemon•garlic mixture over the top, making sure to coat the chicken evenly.

4. Bake for 35•40 minutes, or until the chicken is cooked through and the skin is crispy.

5. Remove the chicken from the oven and sprinkle the crumbled feta cheese over the top.

6. Return the chicken to the oven and bake for an additional 5 minutes, or until the feta is melted.

7. Garnish with chopped fresh parsley before serving.

Nutritional Information (per serving):
Calories: 260
Total Fat: 16g

These Greek•style baked chicken thighs are a delicious and diabetes•friendly main dish. Chicken thighs are a flavorful and affordable cut of meat that is high in protein. The feta cheese and herbs add a Mediterranean twist without adding too many carbs. This dish is low in carbs and high in protein, making it a great option for people with diabetes.

109. Greek•Style Stuffed Artichokes

Ingredient:

• 4 medium artichokes
• 1/4 cup olive oil
• 2 cloves garlic, minced
• 1/2 cup crumbled feta cheese
• 1/4 cup chopped fresh parsley
• 2 tbsp chopped fresh dill
• 1 tsp dried oregano
• 1/4 tsp salt
• 1/4 tsp black pepper
• 1 lemon, cut into wedges

Instructions:

1. Trim the stems of the artichokes and remove the outer leaves until you reach the tender, pale green leaves. Use kitchen shears to snip off the tips of the remaining leaves.

2. In a small bowl, mix together the olive oil, garlic, feta cheese, parsley, dill, oregano, salt, and pepper.

3. Carefully spread open the artichoke leaves and spoon the feta mixture into the center of each artichoke, pressing it down between the leaves.

4. Place the stuffed artichokes in a steamer basket and steam for 30•40 minutes, or until the leaves pull away easily.

5. Serve the stuffed artichokes warm, with lemon wedges on the side.

Nutritional Information (per serving):
Calories: 180
Total Fat: 12g
Saturated Fat: 4g
Cholesterol: 20mg

These Greek•style stuffed artichokes are a delicious and diabetes•friendly appetizer or side dish. Artichokes are a low•carb vegetable that is high in fiber and antioxidants. The feta cheese, herbs, and garlic add a flavorful Mediterranean twist. This dish is a great option for people with diabetes who are looking for a unique and healthy way to enjoy artichokes.

110. Greek•Style Roasted Lamb

Ingredient:

• 3 lb boneless lamb leg roast
• 2 tbsp olive oil
• 3 cloves garlic, minced
• 2 tsp dried oregano
• 1 tsp dried rosemary
• 1/2 tsp salt
• 1/4 tsp black pepper
• 1 lemon, cut into wedges

Instructions:

1. Preheat oven to 375°F. Lightly grease a roasting pan.

2. In a small bowl, mix together the olive oil, garlic, oregano, rosemary, salt, and pepper.

3. Place the lamb roast in the prepared roasting pan. Rub the garlic•herb mixture all over the surface of the lamb.

4. Roast the lamb for 1.5•2 hours, or until it reaches an internal temperature of 145°F for medium•rare, or 160°F for medium.

5. Remove the lamb from the oven and let it rest for 10•15 minutes before slicing.

6. Serve the roasted lamb with lemon wedges on the side.

Nutritional Information (per serving):
Calories: 280
Total Fat: 15g
Saturated Fat: 5g
Cholesterol: 100mg

This Greek•style roasted lamb is a flavorful and tender main dish that is suitable for people with diabetes. Lamb is a lean protein that is high in iron and other essential nutrients. The garlic, oregano, and rosemary add a Mediterranean flair without adding too many carbs. Serve this dish with roasted vegetables or a fresh salad for a complete diabetes•friendly meal.

111. Greek•Style Grilled Eggplant

Ingredient:

• 2 medium eggplants, sliced into 1/2•inch thick rounds
• 2 tbsp olive oil
• 2 tbsp lemon juice
• 2 cloves garlic, minced
• 1 tsp dried oregano
• 1/4 tsp salt
• 1/4 tsp black pepper
• 1/2 cup crumbled feta cheese
• 2 tbsp chopped fresh parsley

Instructions:

1. Preheat grill or grill pan to medium•high heat.

2. In a shallow dish, whisk together the olive oil, lemon juice, garlic, oregano, salt, and pepper.

3. Add the eggplant slices to the dish and toss to coat both sides with the marinade.

4. Grill the eggplant slices for 3•4 minutes per side, or until tender and lightly charred.

5. Transfer the grilled eggplant to a serving platter.

6. Sprinkle the crumbled feta cheese and chopped fresh parsley over the top.

7. Serve warm or at room temperature.

Nutritional Information (per serving):
Calories: 120
Total Fat: 8g
Saturated Fat: 3g
Cholesterol: 15mg

This Greek•style grilled eggplant is a delicious and diabetes•friendly side dish or appetizer. Eggplant is a low•carb vegetable that is high in fiber and antioxidants. The feta cheese and herbs add a Mediterranean flavor without adding too many carbs. This dish is a great option for people with diabetes who are looking for a flavorful and healthy way to enjoy eggplant.

In this journey through the rich and flavorful world of Greek cuisine, we have explored over 110 recipes designed specifically for diabetics. Each dish showcases the vibrant ingredients and traditional methods that make Greek cooking both healthy and delicious. By focusing on fresh vegetables, lean proteins, whole grains, and healthy fats, these recipes offer a balanced approach to managing diabetes without sacrificing taste.

We hope this cookbook has provided you with not only new recipes but also valuable insights into meal planning and nutritional balance. The Mediterranean diet, with its emphasis on whole, natural foods, aligns perfectly with the dietary needs of those managing diabetes. The recipes and tips included aim to help you enjoy your meals while keeping your blood sugar levels in check.

Remember, the key to a successful diabetic diet is consistency and variety. Experiment with different recipes, adapt them to your tastes, and enjoy the process of cooking and eating healthily. With the right resources and a positive approach, managing diabetes through diet can become an enjoyable and fulfilling part of your life.

Thank you for embarking on this culinary adventure with us. We hope that these recipes become staples in your kitchen and that they inspire you to continue exploring the delicious possibilities of diabetic-friendly Greek cooking.